Myths & Facts About Low Speed Collisions and Occupant Injury

by

Dr. Thomas E. Dow

Foreward by Thomas F. Dow D.C.

Dorrance Publishing Co
585 Alpha Drive
Pittsburgh, PA 15238
Visit our website at www.dorrancebookstore.com

ISBN: 979-8-88925-359-4
eISBN: 979-8-88925-859-9

Dedication

"The author of *Low-Speed Collisions and Soft Tissue Injury* is Dr. Thomas E. Dow, a chiropractor in New York that has over 40 years of experience in the treatment of traumatic injuries dealing with the musculoskeletal system. He is my father, and throughout my life it's become clear how much he does to help others. He has always strived to teach me that success is not measured in how many material items one may have, but it's measured in your own idea of success and how many people's lives you changed once you retire from earth. His willingness to teach people things comes from an early age when he learned about chiropractic from another chiropractor. Also, he was also a high school teacher who taught science curriculum. In the mid 1980's and early 1990's he gained vast experience and education in dealing with patients involved in motor vehicle accidents. I remember as a child going to these convention centers full of personal injury attorneys. There he was, up on the podium teaching them about soft tissue injuries such as whiplash and how it is important to know about the mechanism of the injury. At the time I thought it was very boring and couldn't wait to get out and go do something else. Now later on in life, I realize how important it was that he was there doing all that hard work. My father and I are currently business partners and own several successful practices on Long Island. When I first became a chiropractor it was amazing when I found out how many people knew my father and remembered the seminars and lectures he gave. It was almost like he was a celebrity in the personal injury arena. His drive and willingness to keep going stronger and stronger each day is mind-blowing. This book that you are about to read is one of his most prized lifetime accomplishments, I've heard it time and time again, "before I leave this planet I am going to write a book and it will be a best seller". Well, I guess now the book is complete, we will see what happens next. Good luck dad and I love you so much."

Introduction

For many years I have been treating patients with injuries, many of which are from motor vehicle accidents. Most of these patients respond well, but the great majority of them continue to suffer to some extent for the rest of their lives. In other words, they are never the same as they were before the accident. I've spent years researching and lecturing about motor vehicle accidents and soft tissue injury and have finally come to understand why patients continue to suffer.

Soft Tissue Injury and Attorneys

I have found that most of the time personal injury attorneys are excited when they have a hard tissue injury client knock on their door, and not so excited when a soft tissue injury client knocks on their door. The reason for this is because hard tissue injuries such as fractures are easy to visualize and prove (i.e.: x ray or CAT scan) whereas soft tissue injury historically has been much more difficult to visualize and prove. As a matter of fact, I have known many personal injury attorneys that will not even take a soft tissue injury case.

The Truth

In my forty years of practice, I have found that soft tissue injury is usually more serious than fractures and produces future pain, suffering, and degenerative changes for the rest of the patient's life. Of course, there are always exceptions to this where hard tissue injuries are more serious, but this is not usually the case.

When I lecture, one of the first questions I ask my audience is, "If you've ever broken a bone in your life, please raise your hand." Let's say twenty-five people put up their hands. I then ask those who raised their hands, "Please put your hand back up if you still have pain and weakness at the fracture site or if the fracture site causes you any decreased function." Maybe one or two people put their hands back up.

I then ask the following question. "If you've ever injured your knee, ankle, shoulder, elbow, wrist, spine, or other joint of our body without causing a fracture and you were told you had a sprain, strain, muscle or ligament tear, or any other kind of soft tissue injury, please raise your hand." Let's say twenty-five people put up their hands. I then ask them to raise their hand again if they still have pain, weakness, or decreased function at that body part that was injured, and the majority of the audience puts their hands back up again.

So as can be seen from the above, soft tissue injuries produce much more lasting pain, suffering, and disability than most hard tissue injuries, and usually ends up creating an arthritic joint in the future.

The Goal

The goal that I have in this publication is to inform the reader, in a true or false format, about the myths and facts about auto collisions and the prognosis for the injuries that are produced as a result.

The Test

The next section of this publication is a twenty-four question true or false test that I would like each reader to take BEFORE they read the answers. Let's see how many you get right and how many you get wrong after reading. Good Luck.

Accident Questionnaire

At the end of this publication an Accident Questionnaire. I strongly encourage its use by both health care providers and personal injury attorneys. This will give the user a better understanding of what had transpired with the occupant at the time of the collision and afterward.

Motor Vehicle Accident Facts and Myths

1) Minimal vehicle damage causes minimal passenger injury. True False

2) With a five miles-per-hour rear end impact, the person's head moves back and then forward at five miles per hour. With a twenty-five miles per hour impact the person's head moves a little faster. True False

3) The best seat position that produces the least amount of injury to an occupant in a rear end collision is with the seat angled back so the occupant's head is further back and braced on the seat for impact. True False

4) The best headrest position for an occupant that produces the least injury is with the headrest above the top of the head. True False

5) If a vehicle is stopped on an icy road and is rear ended, there will be less injury to the occupant of the vehicle that is being struck when it slides forward after the collision because the vehicle is being pushed away and will have minimal damage. True False

6) Temporal mandibular joint (TMJ) injury is very common to an occupant of a vehicle after a rear end collision. True False

7) Wearing a seatbelt prevents lower back injury from rear end collisions. True False

8) The car that is hit from behind accelerates after impact faster if the rear vehicle has a greater mass. True False

9) Some occupants may not feel symptoms from a motor vehicle accident for weeks or even months later. True False

10) After a soft tissue injury occurs and instability occurs in the joint, arthritic changes always happen afterward. True False

11) At least twenty-one days must elapse before an EMG/NCV is performed. True False

12) After a spinal nerve root is compressed by a herniated disc, muscle weakness occurs before numbness develops. True False

13) A stand-up MRI study will always show the same result as a laying down MRI. True False

14) You must wait at least thirty days before an MRI is performed after a motor vehicle accident. True False

15) An infant seated in the rear seat facing backward has a low chance of developing a neck injury in a rear end collision. True False

16) If an occupant sees the sees the rear end collision about to happen in his/her rear-view mirror, the best thing the occupant can do is to lean forward away from the seatback and reach across to hold his/her child against the seat back of the child's seat. True False

17) If after a rear end collision, the vehicle being struck hits another vehicle in front of him/her, there will be less injury to the occupants in the rear-ended vehicle because the vehicle will travel less distance forward. True False

18) Seatbelts prevent all injuries in a rear end collision. True False

19) A rear lap belt harness can cause lumbar spine fractures. True False

20) Some occupants have suffered carotid artery dissections and strokes after being rear ended. True False

21) A whiplash victim can suffer from neck pain which radiates down the arm to the hand and have normal x ray findings, normal MRI findings, and a positive examination demonstrating a radiculopathy. True False

22) A person with a pre-existing lumbar disc condition will be injured less than a person without a pre-existing lumbar spine condition. True False

23) In general, fractures cause much more long-term effects than sprains. True False

24) You can't get a concussion or traumatic brain injury during an accident unless you strike your head. True False

1) Minimal vehicle damage causes minimal occupant injury.

Answer: FALSE

The amount of damage to a vehicle after an accident is sometimes not related to the amount of injury to an occupant. As a matter of fact, many times there is an inverse relationship to vehicle damage and occupant injury.

Let's look at the two following scenarios:

1) A vehicle is cemented into the road (target vehicle) and cannot move on rear impact (by the bullet vehicle). When the target vehicle is struck from behind by the bullet vehicle, the energy of momentum of the bullet vehicle will be transferred to the target vehicle by crushing, damage and absorption of this energy. The bullet vehicle also gets crushed by some of this momentum. In collision reconstruction this is called an inelastic collision (plastic collision). This is a physics law called the conservation of momentum. All of this energy is transferred as crushing of both vehicles. This creates a lot of damage to both vehicles. The target vehicle does not move so the occupants in the vehicle do not move. Therefore, if the occupants don't move, there is no whiplash or any other injuries to the occupants because they don't move. (Unless of course a part of the debris or a part of the deformed vehicle strikes the occupants from the inside.)

2) A vehicle is stopped on an icy declined road (target vehicle) and is struck from behind by a bullet vehicle. At impact the target vehicle accelerates forward very rapidly because there is limited friction with the tire and the road. The target vehicle doesn't have much

time to crush and sustain damage because it is rapidly pushed away from the bullet vehicle. In collision reconstruction this is called an **ELASTIC COLLISION.** Therefore, there is minimal damage to the target vehicle. The bullet vehicle continues to move forward down the declined icy road after impact. In this case the occupants in the target vehicle immediately are thrown back against the seat, they slide up the seat (ramping) and their head whips back forcefully and rapidly and then when the vehicle comes to a stop is forced forward rapidly (This is called whiplash or acceleration/deceleration injury) In this scenario, the occupants are seriously injured because they have moved quickly inside the vehicle, and there is minimal damage to the vehicle.

The speed of impact and the weight of the vehicles will obviously be important factors in every situation described above.

So we must look at occupant movement after collisions and not the amount of damage to a vehicle in determining how seriously injured an occupant becomes after a collision.

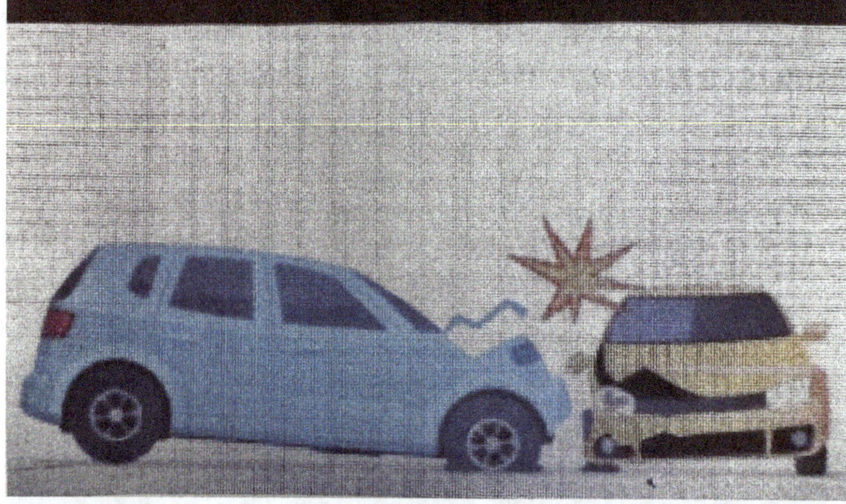
INELASTIC COLLISION

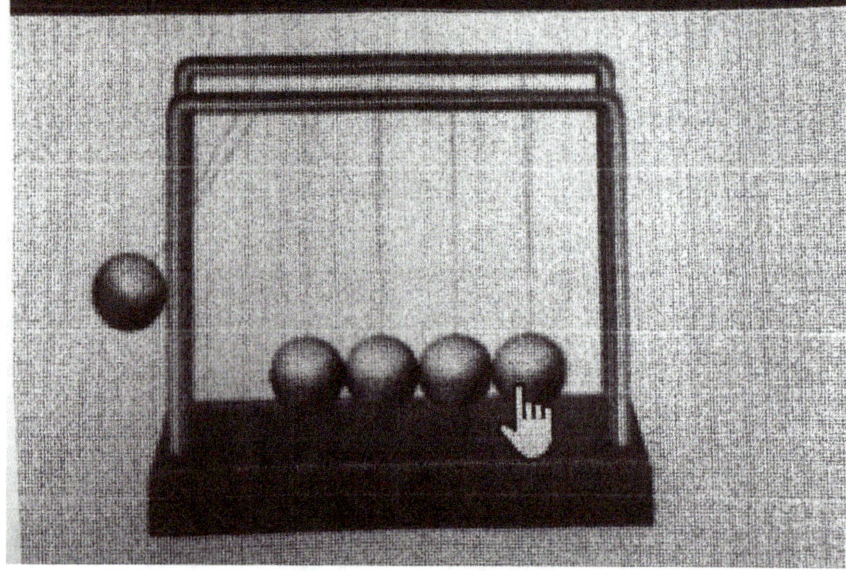
ELASTIC COLLISION

2) With a five miles per hour rear end impact, the occupant's head moves back five miles per hour and then forward five miles per hour. With a twenty-five miles per hour rear end impact, the occupant's head moves back and forth a little faster. FALSE

(McConnell et al., 1993, States et al., (1969), Weissner and Enssien, 1985)

When a vehicle is rear ended the occupant's head moves back and forth two and a half to five times the speed of impact. This is why this movement is called whiplash or acceleration/deceleration motion. Imagine the movement of a whip. When the handle of a whip is moved back and then forward, the top of the whip moves back and forth much faster than the handle. This same motion occurs when a person suffers from a whiplash injury.

So a rear end collision with a five miles per hour impact could cause the occupant's head to move back and forth at twelve and a half to twenty-five miles per hour. With a twenty miles per hour impact, the occupant's head could move fifty to one hundred miles per hour. The skull weighs approximately eleven pounds and sits on top of seven small bones called vertebra that are connected to each other by ligaments, muscles, and discs. With this rapid movement back and forth, it's easy to understand how these ligaments, discs, and muscles can be easily injured in a low impact rear end collision.

(Mertz HJ Jr, Patrick LM: Investigation of the kinematics and kinetics of whiplash, Severy DM, Mathewson JH, Bechtol CO: Controlled automobile rear-end collisions-an investigation of related engineering and medical phenomenon, Foreman SH, Croft AC Whiplash Injuries: The Cervical Acceleration/ Deceleration Syndrome, Baltimore, Williams & Wilkins, 1988.)

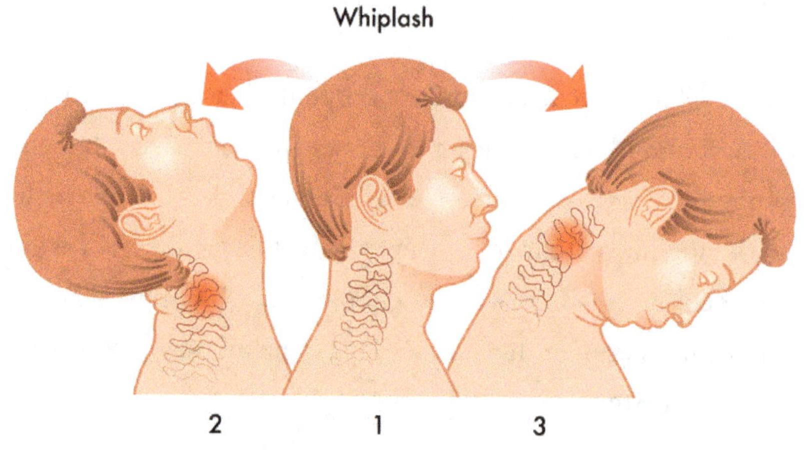

3) The best seat position that produces the least injury to an occupant in a rear end collision is with the seat angled back so the occupant's head is further back and braced on the seat and headrest. FALSE

Research with crash dummies has shown that the first movement that occurs to an occupant after a rear end collision is the following: The occupant actually slides up the seat. The seat is literally pushed forward from underneath him/her to make this upward sliding occur. This phenomenon is called ramping.

If the seat back is vertically straight up and down, the ramping will be minimal. The more the seat back is angled back the more sliding up the seat will occur. There are members of the younger generations that think it is cool when they drive with seat back angled far back and they hold the steering wheel with one straight arm. It may look cool but it's actually very dangerous. There have been rear end collisions in which occupants have actually been thrown through the rear window of the vehicle due to this angled back seat back position.

So, try to keep your seat back upright as much as possible to avoid ramping in a rear end collision.

(Occupant kinematics in a high speed vehicle to vehicle rear end collision, International Journal of Vehicle Safety Vol 12, No 2

Sung-Woo & Jingwen H, Mertz HJ Jr. Patrick LM: Investigation of the kinematics and kinetics of whiplash. In: Proceedings, 11th Stapp Car Crash Conference, SAE 670919. Detroit, MI Society of Automotive Engineers, 1967.

Croft AC: Biomechanics. In: Foreman SM, Croft AC (eds): Whiplash Injuries: The Cervical Acceleration/ Deceleration Syndrome. Baltimore, Williams & Wilkins Co., 1988, pp 53-72)

4) The best headrest position that produces the least amount of occupant injury in a rear end collision is with the headrest above the top of the head. **TRUE**

When an occupant is rear ended in a motor vehicle the first motion of the occupant is to move up or ramp up the seat back. The next motion is for the occupant's head to rapidly accelerate back into extension. If the headrest is above the head before this ramping occurs, by the time the occupant slides up the seat, the headrest is positioned behind the occupant's head, thus preventing further extension and also preventing more injury.

If the headrest is positioned below or behind the occupant's head before impact, after impact the occupant slides or ramps up the seatback and when the head goes back into extension, the headrest now is behind the neck, and the headrest acts like a karate chop. This causes even more hyperextension of the neck and more injury.

There are some vehicles that don't even have headrests such as some vans and trucks. Most buses don't have headrests either. There are also some vehicles that have seat backs that go higher up in place of headrests that may not be high enough to stop the extension of the neck after ramping and rear impact.

So when you get back in your car, make sure you move your headrest up to the top of your head.

(Occupant kinematics in a high speed vehicle to vehicle rear end collision, International Journal of Vehicle Safety Vol 12, No 2, Sung-Woo & Jingwen H, Mertz HJ Jr. Patrick LM: Investigation of the kinematics and kinetics of whiplash. In: Proceedings, 11th Stapp Car Crash Conference, SAE 670919. Detroit, MI Society of Automotive Engineers, 1967.

Croft AC: Biomechanics. In: Foreman SM, Croft AC (eds): Whiplash Injuries: The Cervical Acceleration/ Deceleration Syndrome. Baltimore, Williams & Wilkins Co., 1988, pp 53-72)

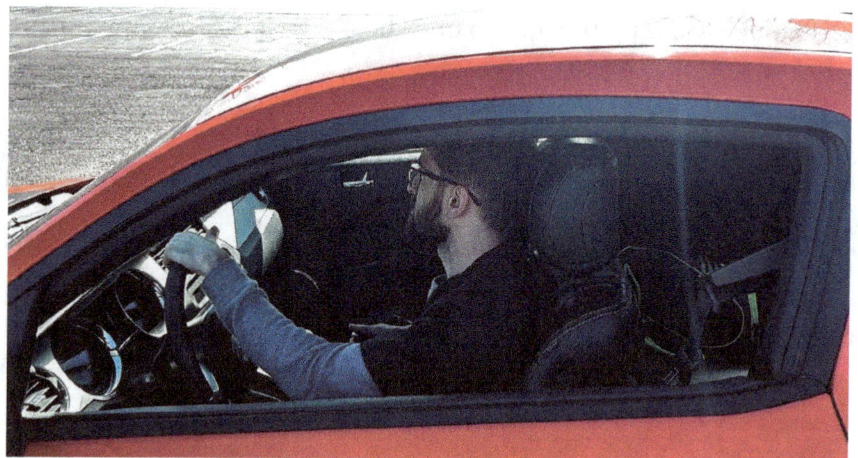

Just a quick head's up!

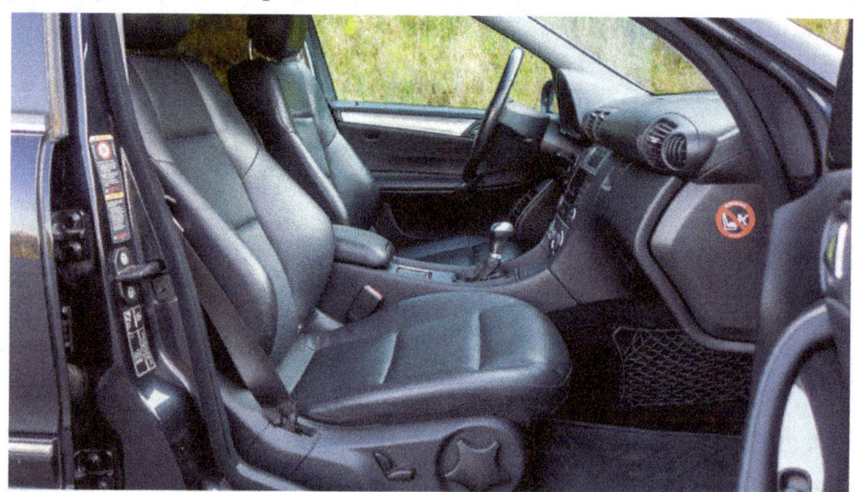

5) If a vehicle is stopped on an icy road and is rear ended, there is less injury to the occupant of the vehicle that is being struck when it slides forward after the collision because the vehicle is being pushed away and will have minimal damage. FALSE

The most important thing to remember about occupant injury after a collision is to understand what the occupant was doing inside the vehicle, the position they were in and how they moved inside the vehicle after collision. The amount of damage a vehicle has after a collision DOES NOT determine how injured an occupant becomes! In the collision above, when the vehicle slides forward, the vehicle is basically pushed underneath the occupant causing the occupant to ramp or slide up the seat and then sustaining a serious whiplash injury. When the vehicle slides away because there is little friction between the road and the vehicle's tires, the vehicle being hit has little time to crush and sustain a lot of damage and the vehicle doing the hitting continues to slide forward with the vehicle that it hit.

Other factors will also determine if and how a vehicle that is being hit will move.

The following conditions will cause less acceleration after collision: Inclination of the road, the occupant's foot firmly on the brake, dry road conditions.

The following conditions will cause greater acceleration after collision: Declination of the road, the occupant's foot off the brake, and slippery road conditions.

Taking the above into consideration, the occupants may sustain more injury in the vehicle they are occupying if the vehicle is moving forward before the rear impact because the foot is off the brake.

Also it is very important to understand what the occupants were doing inside the vehicle before impact. Is the occupant leaning forward to change a radio station or adjust the volume? Is the occupant reaching to the passenger's seat to pick something up? Is the occupant turning the heat up because it is too cold? Is the occupant texting? Is the occupant looking and handing the baby in the car seat a toy? Is the occupant checking their makeup in the rear-view mirror? Is the occupant having a sip of coffee or a bite of a sandwich?

All of these actions will produce different body parts injured after collision so it's important for the doctor to understand these dynamics.

(Anderson RA, Welcher JB, Szabo TJ, Eubanks JJ, Haight WR "Effects of Braking on Human Occupant and Vehicle Kinematics in Low Speed Rear-End Collisions", Society of Automotive Engineers, (SAE No. 980298), pp 1-13, 1998

Robbins MS: "Lack of Relationship Between Vehicle Damage and Occupant Injury", Society of Automotive Engineers, SP-1226, (SAE No. 970494). Pp 117-119, 1988)

Roberts VL, Compton CP, "The relationship Between Delta V and Injury". Proceedings of the 37th Stapp Car Crash Conference (SAE

NO. 933111), pp 35-41, 1993

Romily DP, Thomson RW, Navin FPD, MacNabb MJ: Low Speed Impacts and the Elastic Properties of Automobiles." 12th International Technical Conference on Experimental Safety Vehicles, pp 1199-1205, 1989)

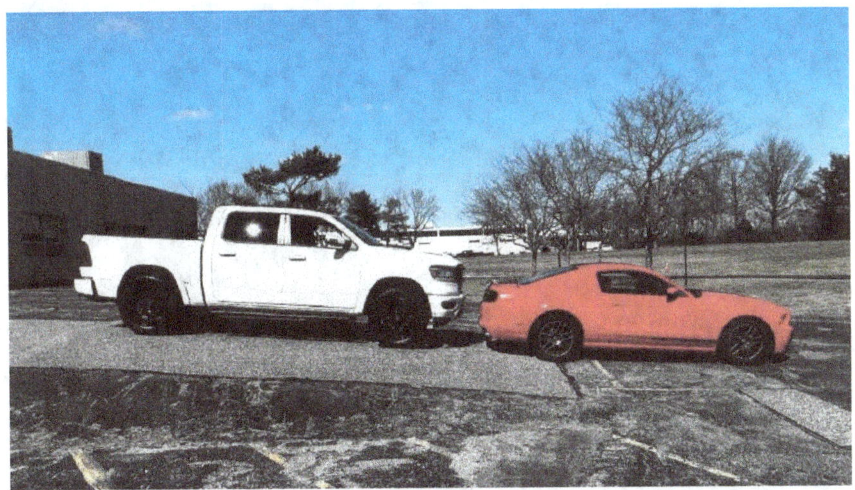

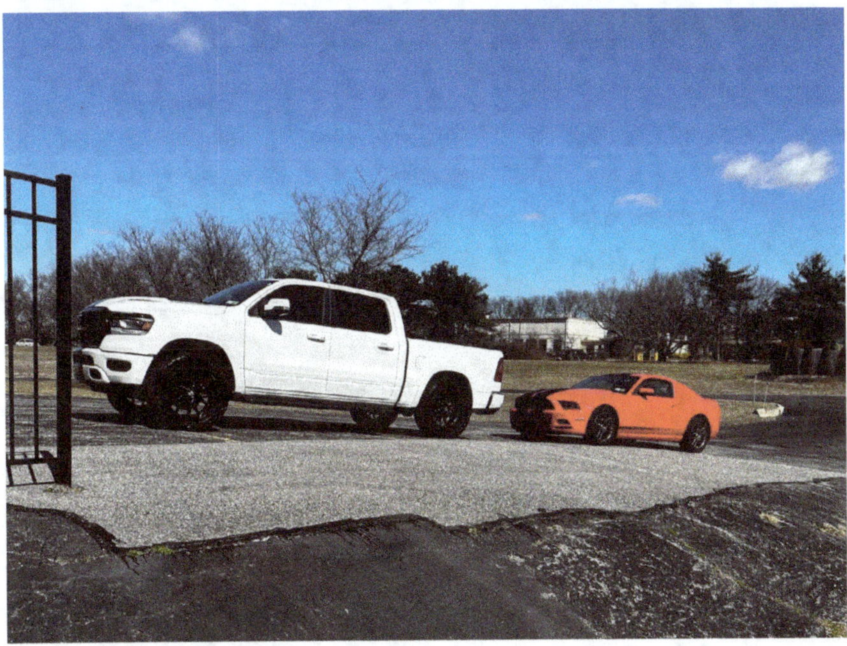

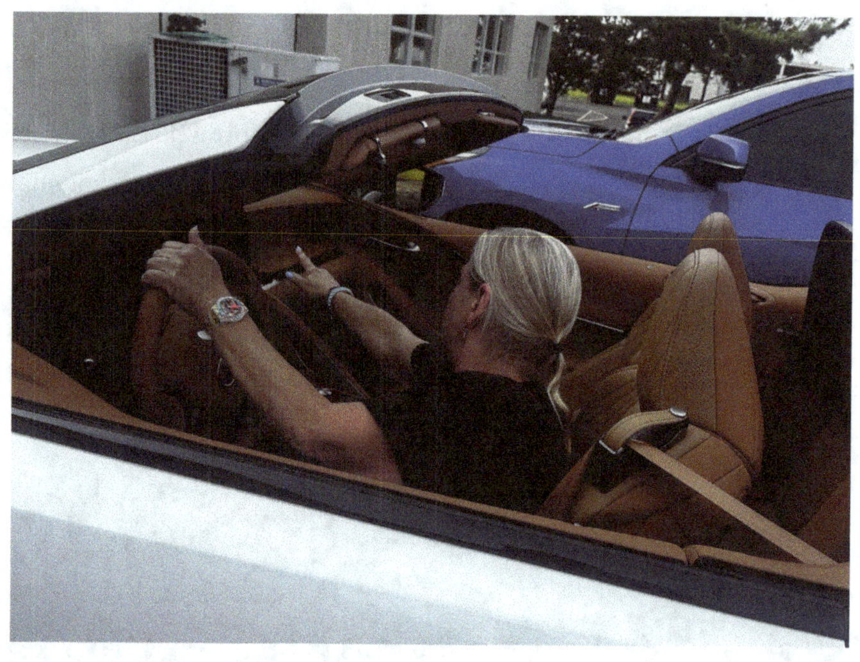

6) Temporomandibular Joint (TMJ) injury is very common to an occupant of a vehicle after a rear end collision. TRUE

After a vehicle is struck from behind the occupant slides up the seat back, the head is thrown backward, the neck goes into extension and the jaw is forced open. After the vehicle comes to stop, the neck flies forward into flexion and the jaw snaps shut rapidly. Occupants have actually broken teeth with this rapid opening and closing, but this is the lesser of the injury that can occur.

The jaw opens and closes at a joint called the temporomandibular joint (TMJ). The TMJ is a synovial, condylar, and hinge-type joint. The joint involves fibrocartilaginous surfaces and an articular disc which divides the joint into two cavities. These superior and inferior articular cavities are lined by separate superior and inferior synovial membranes. When the TMJ opens and snaps back quickly, structures can be easily torn and ripped. The disc can actually become ripped and displaced and sometimes the jaw becomes locked which prevents normal opening and closing of the mouth. One can also see the mandible (lower jaw) move to the left and right abnormally when opening and closing the mouth.

This abnormal motion and symptoms are often referred to as TMD or Temporomandibular disorder. The following symptoms can occur as a result:

Jaw pain

Headaches

Earaches

Pain in the neck or shoulders

Difficulty opening your mouth wide

Jaws that "lock" in the open- or closed-mouth position

Clicking, popping, or grating sounds in the jaw joint when opening or closing your mouth

A tired feeling in your face

Difficulty chewing

Tinnitus, or ringing in your ears

Changes in the way your teeth fit together

Swelling on the side of your face

Tooth pain

It is important to assess for this in all whiplash injuries. If a TMJ injury has occurred there are a variety of different treatment approaches, but it must first be identified by the practitioner.

Here are some widely used treatment for TMD:

Physical therapy

Dental appliances to wear at night to relax the facial muscles and to prevent grinding of the teeth and pressure on the TMJ.

Posture changes: sitting up straight as opposed to slouching helps puts less stress on the TMJ, sleeping on your back as opposed to your side creates less pressure on the TMJ, not chewing hard objects or gum decreases stress on the TMJ.

Surgery as a last resort.

Uncorrected TMD can lead to many painful years and arthritis in the future caused by this abnormal opening and closing.
(Croft AC: The cervical acceleration/deceleration syndrome. In: Steigerwald DP, Croft AC (eds): Whiplash and Temporomandibular Joint Dysfunction: an Interdisciplinary Approach to Case Management, Encinitas, Keiser Publishing Co., 1992.)

Charles E. Fernandez, DC, MAppSe, Abid Amiri, DC, Joseph Jaime, DC, Paul Delaney, DC, PhD: The relationship of whiplash injury to temporomandibular joint disorders: a narrative literature review. J Chiropractic Medicine 2005-Dec; 8(4): 171-186)

It is important to evaluate for this disorder whenever a person suffers a whiplash injury.

TMJ DISORDER

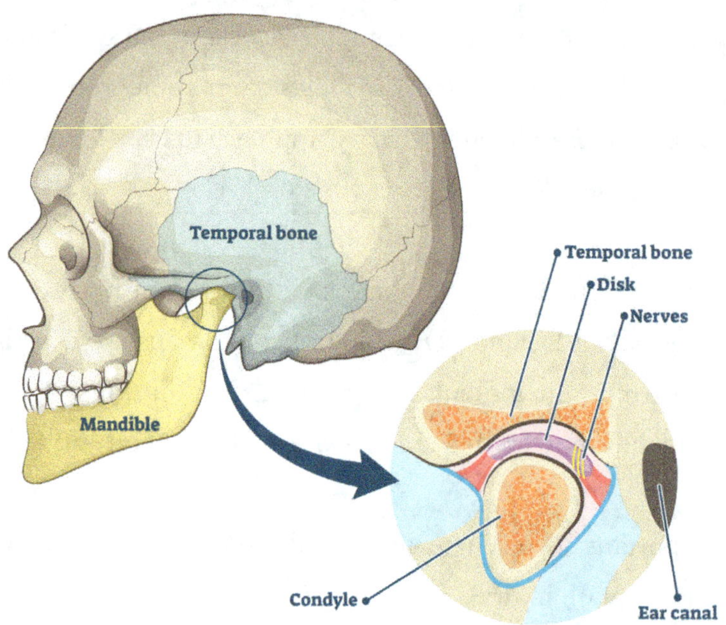

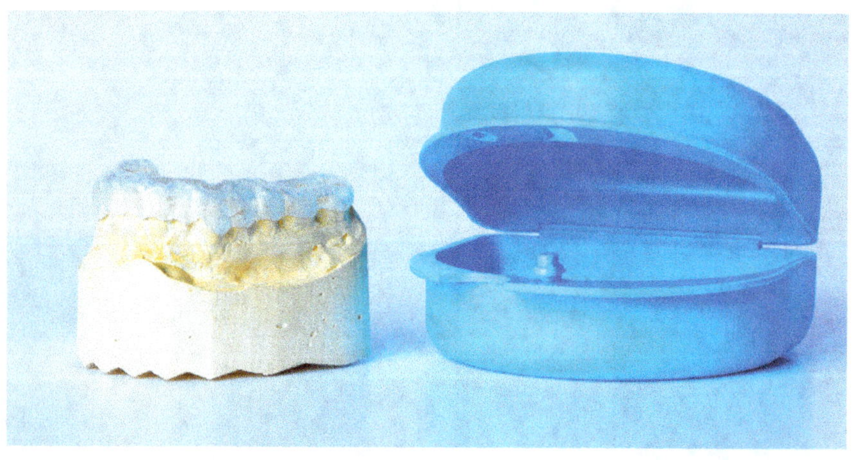

7) Wearing a seatbelt prevents lower back injury from rear end collisions.

FALSE

When a driver is rear ended in a motor vehicle accident, the driver moves or ramps up the seat, then the head extends rapidly backwards at two and a half to five times the speed of impact. Then as the vehicle comes to an abrupt stop the head rapidly moves forward as does the right shoulder as the left shoulder is restrained by the three-point seat belt system.

This twisting rapid forward movement causes injury to the lumbar spine and can easily cause lower back injury. Authors Croft and Foreman report that fifty percent of acceleration/deceleration (CAD) injuries have an associated low back injury.

In racing boats and race cars, there is usually a four-point restraint system in which the seatbelt restrains both shoulders, thus preventing the whole body and both shoulders from moving forward in a frontal or rear end collision.

Three-point seatbelt systems can cause many other types of injuries when the body twists and moves forward. Some of these injuries are abdominal, shoulder, pelvic, bladder, and hip amongst others.

If one is unlucky enough to wear only a lapbelt, lumbar spine fractures and dislocations have occurred. Also many times the seatbelt is worn improperly which can cause even more serious injuries.

Maybe someday all cars will be equipped with four-point restraint systems.

(Holt BW: Spines and Seat belts: mechanisms of spinal injury in motor vehicle crashes. Med J Austral 2:411-413, 1976

Johnson DL, Falci S: The diagnosis and treatment of pediatric lumbar spine injuries caused by rear seat lap belts. Neurosurg 26(3)434-440,1990.

Huelke D, Kaufer H: Vertebral column injuries and seat belts. J Trauma 15:304-318, 1975

Rutledge R, Thomason M, Oller D, Meredith W, Moylan J, Clancy T, Cunningham P, Baker C: The spectrum of abdominal injuries associated with the use of seat belts. J Trauma 31(6): 820-826, 1991.

Asbun HJ, Irani H, Roe EJ, Bloch JH: Intra-abdominal seat belt injury. J Trauma 30(2): 189-193, 1990 .)

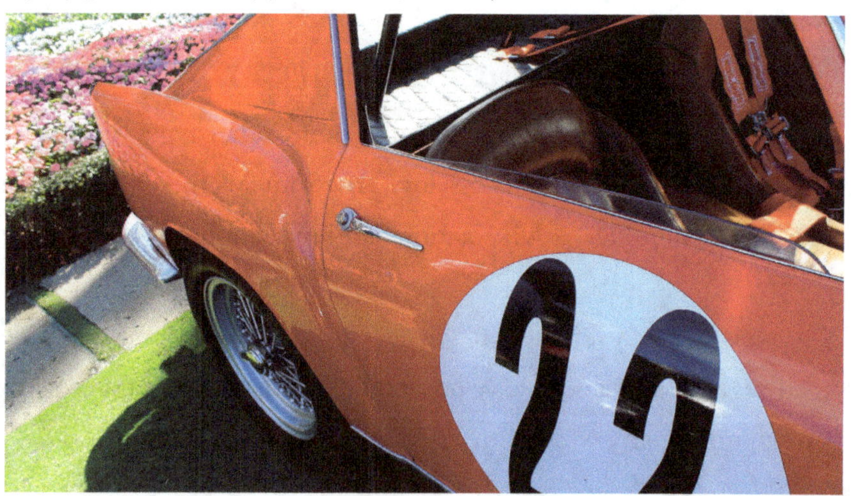

8) The car that is hit from behind accelerates after impact faster if the striking vehicle has a greater mass. TRUE

There is a law in physics called The Law of Conservation of Linear Momentum. This law states that when no external forces act on a system of two colliding objects, the vector sum of their linear momentum remains constant and is unaffected by their mutual interaction. So the sum of the momentum must remain the same.

Momentum is equal to mass times velocity. P-momentum, M-Mass, V- Velocity

P-MxV

So the more an object weighs and the faster it moves, the greater the momentum.

So if a barge strikes a dock at two miles per hour it will create tremendous damage to the dock because of its mass and subsequent momentum.

If a bullet hits a wall at two miles per hour, with its low mass, it has a very low momentum and will create no damage to the wall. However, if the bullet is traveling at two hundred miles per hour and hits a wall, it will do a lot of damage because of its speed and subsequent high momentum.

When a stationary object is struck by a moving object with a certain momentum, the object which is being struck will have this momentum transferred to it.

If a car is stopped and weighs three thousand pounds, and it is struck by a vehicle of the same weight that is traveling at thirty miles per hour, the following momentum equations will apply:

Vehicle 1 (Target): Mass=3000lbs x velocity= 0 mph has zero momentum. Vehicle 2 (Bullet): Mass 3000 lbs x velocity-30 mph has 90,000 units of momentum. So after collision, for momentum to be conserved, if vehicle #1 (Target) is pushed away and the striking vehicle #2 (Bullet) stops immediately after the collision, the vehicle #1 must move away at thirty miles per hour. (Assuming there is no friction on the road and there is no crushing or damage to this vehicle. Remember vehicle damage and crushing uses up momentum and dissipates some of the energy and momentum)

If the striking vehicle (Bullet Vehicle) is heavier (ie: a truck), the following equation may occur:

Vehicle 1: Mass=3000lbs x velocity= 0 mph has zero momentum
Vehicle 2: Mass 15,000 lbs x velocity=30 mph has 450,000 units of momentum

Mass of vehicles (10)

A streetcar traveling at a speed of 3 mph will produce the same damage as a compact car traveling at 40mph.

So after collision for momentum to be conserved, if the stopped vehicle is pushed away and the striking vehicle stops after the collision, the vehicle moving away must move away at one hundred fifty miles per hour. (Again, assuming there is no friction on the road and there is no crushing or damage to this vehicle. Remember vehicle damage and crushing uses up momentum and dissipates some of the energy and momentum)

The main point is that the more massive the vehicle in the rear is (Bullet vehicle) the faster the stopped vehicle (Target vehicle) accelerates after collision and the more injured the occupants become because the occupants are moving faster inside the vehicle!

To truly understand the injuries which may have occurred to an occupant that has been involved in an automobile accident, all of the factors above are important and must be considered. These are very important questions that you must ask you occupant when trying to examine and assess injuries caused by a motor vehicle collision.

(Szabo, TJ, Rusty Haight, WR, Welcher, JB: "Analysis of Low Speed Collisions" 1998)

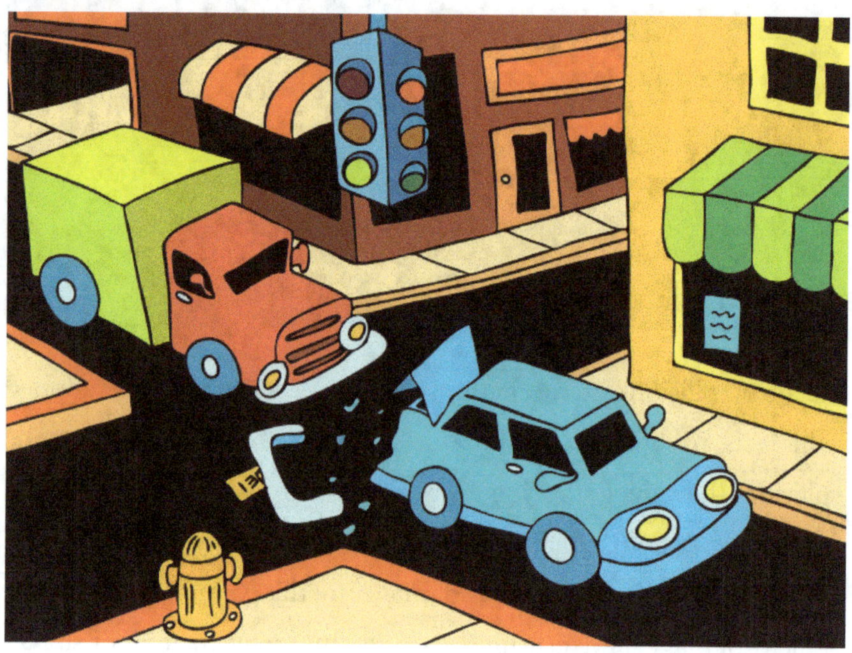

9) Some occupants may not feel symptoms from a motor vehicle accident for weeks or even months later. TRUE

Dr. Nicholas Gotten, in an article published in the Journal of the American Medical Association, says that there can be several days delay in the onset of symptoms.

Dr.'s Braff & Rosner report in the New York State Medical Journal that sometimes months or even years may elapse before symptoms develop.

The reason for this delay is that once soft tissues are injured, swelling and inflammation sometimes take time to develop which then causes symptoms. As a perfect example of this, I'm sure you have had the experience of getting a splinter, and sometimes you don't even know that you've gotten it until the inflammation and swelling starts sometimes days later. Or you may feel a pinch, and then look to see if you have a splinter and can't see anything. Eventually your body will react and recognize that this is a foreign body and days or weeks later try to push this foreign body out of your body. You might notice redness (inflammation), then maybe a bump and some puss (white blood cells trying to prevent infection), and then you squeeze it and out comes the splinter.

This is why a complete and thorough initial examination after a trauma is crucial following a motor vehicle accident. The examiner must check the patient to make sure the patient just hasn't felt the injury yet because enough inflammation hasn't happened yet.

Another phenomenon called neurological gating can occur with trauma. If an occupant has multiple areas of injury, he/she may only be aware of the areas of ones producing the most pain and barely feel or not feel at all the other injured areas. This occurs because of the neurological gating mechanism. At the spinal cord level there is a gating mechanism (a reflex loop) that will either allow pain signals to go up to the brain or it can block the signals to the brain, opening and closing the gate. As a protective mechanism it is theorized that this has been evolutionarily developed to make us aware of the most intense pain signals first while blocking out the least intense pain signals. A perfect example of this is the following: let's make believe that tomorrow morning you wake up with mild lower back pain. You get out of bed, walk toward the bathroom and bump into a hundred-pound box you left on the counter the night before. The box falls to the ground and lands right on top pf your foot. All of a sudden your back pain disappears and all you can feel is the pain in your foot. This is because of this gating mechanism taking place in your nervous system without you even being aware of it. Your body is trying to protect you and make you aware of the most dangerous signals in your environment.

So when examining a patient that has suffered a trauma such as a motor vehicle accident it is paramount that the whole body is examined. I have often had spoken with patients that have been in motor vehicle accidents who have only complained of neck pain and lower back pain on initial consultation. When I examine them, I examine the whole person. I bring their shoulders, elbows, wrists, hips, knees, and ankles through their normal ranges of motion and palpate all of these structures and many times a patient will jump and say, "ouch, I didn't even know that that hurt."

Also when the most injured body part starts to get better, and the pain in this area lessens, other areas may begin to hurt. In the case of the box being dropped on the foot, when the foot starts to heal and the pain lessens, all of a sudden the lower back pain begins to return. This is not because the lower back condition got better as a result of having a heavy box dropped on the foot, but because the neurological gate has become open again allowing the pain signals from the lower back to get to the brain.

It is common for a patient that has been in a motor vehicle accident to sometimes weeks or months later start to report symptoms that weren't there right after the accident. This is due to the gating reasons described above but also due to compensations in gait and activities of daily living caused by the person's initial injuries.

Let's say for example someone injures their knee and ankle in an auto accident and has to use crutches, braces, and maybe even have surgery. For weeks this person will have to be getting around with a very abnormal gait which may cause a disc herniation in the lumbar spine. Or a person may have a shoulder injury and need to wear a sling for a prolonged time period which puts pressure on the neck which may cause a neck injury. Or a person may have a lower back injury with sciatica which may cause them to limp thus causing a torn meniscus in their knee. All of these scenarios are possible, and I have seen them happen in practice over the last forty years.

This is why it is also imperative that the treating doctor continually examine and monitor the patient as he/she moves through a course of treatment. It is also from a med legal standpoint to document all that happens during the course of treatment after a motor vehicle collision.

(Gotten N: Survey of one hundred cases of whiplash injury after settlement of litigation. JAMA 162 (9): 865-867, 1956

Braaf MM, Rosner S: Symptomatology and treatment of injuries of the neck. NY State J Med 55:237-242, 1955)

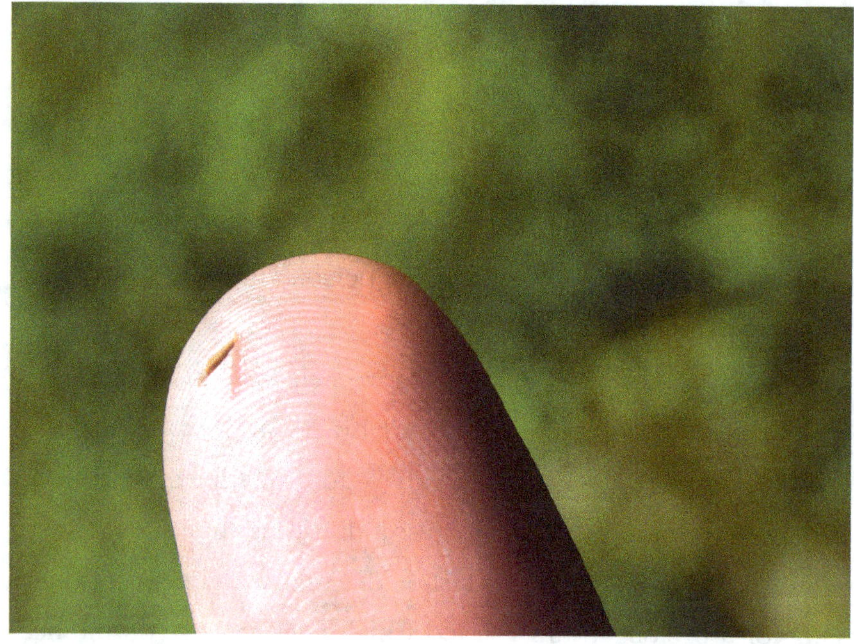

10) After a soft tissue injury occurs and instability occurs in the joint, arthritic changes always happen afterward. **TRUE**

When a soft tissue injury occurs in a joint, ligaments, muscles and tendons can be injured, stretched or torn. A ligament is a structure that holds two bones together. A tendon is the end of a muscle and usually attaches to bone. These structures are meant to keep joints stable and aligned in our bodies keeping the joints strong. When a football player is hit and tears his ACL (Anterior Cruciate Ligament), his knee becomes unstable. The ACL prevents the femur from sliding forward on the tibia. If this ligament is stretched out and not repaired, with every step taken, the femur slides forward on the tibia. After continued abnormal stress on this joint, the cartilage between the knee will wear out and calcium will be deposited in the area in the body's attempt to stabilize the joint (osteoarthritis).

It's similar to what happens to the front tires of your car. If the front end of your car is out of alignment, eventually one side of the front tires will wear out prematurely.

The human body is no different. Dr. Ehni and Dr. J. Wickstrom report that chronic instability leads to disc degeneration which results in spondylosis or arthritic conditions. These same changes also occur in any other joint of the body that has become unstable due to soft tissue injury. So, for example, a person with soft tissue injury to the knee, with resultant instability will end up with degeneration of the knee with arthritic changes.

The reason why these soft these soft tissue injuries to muscles and ligaments are as follows. Dr.'s Croft & Foreman and Dr. Gunn report that muscles heal with collagen scar tissue and that this scar tissue is weaker and less elastic than normal tissue and are supersensitive. They also report that ligaments heal poorly and incompletely due to poor blood supply which is why the resultant instability is usually permanent in nature.

So every time an occupant sustains a soft tissue injury to a joint which results in instability (and almost all do) arthritic changes and degeneration are what the future holds for this joint.

There have been many times in practice over the last forty years that I have had a patient come in to my office complaining of, for instance, neck pain. I ask the patient if they have ever had any trauma to their neck and they say no. After examination and x ray I find that there are one or two vertebral segments which have a lot of degeneration and the rest of the cervical spine is normal. On further questioning of the patient, I ask, "are you sure you never injured your neck previously, maybe many years ago?" Always the patient remembers the time that they had neck pain maybe after a wrestling match when he was in high school or a skiing injury where he had neck pain for a few days and then the pain went away, etc. So what had happened was that after the injury many years prior, the vertebral segments became unstable because of the ligaments and other soft tissues which were torn or stretched out, and the result was instability of the normal motion of the vertebra for many years causing the discs to wear out and calcium being deposited in its place. This is called degenerative (osteo) arthritis.

(Ehni G: Degenerative motion segment encroachments. In: Cervical Arthrosis: Diseases of the Cervical Motion Segments. Chicago, Year Book, 1984, p 54

Wickstom J: Effects of whiplash injury. JAMA 194:40, 1965)

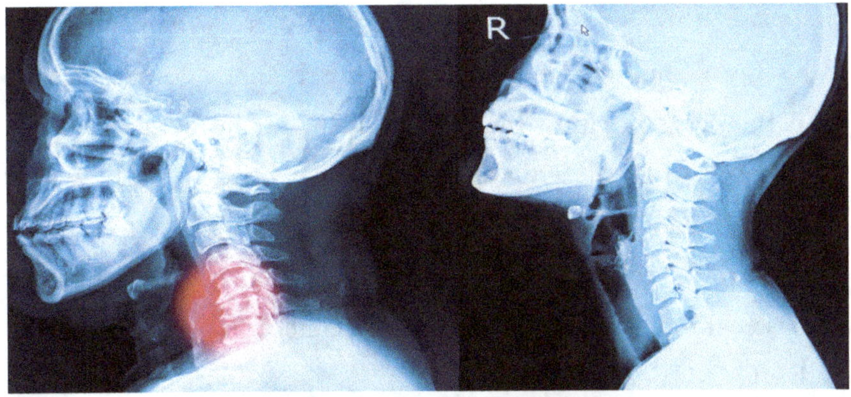

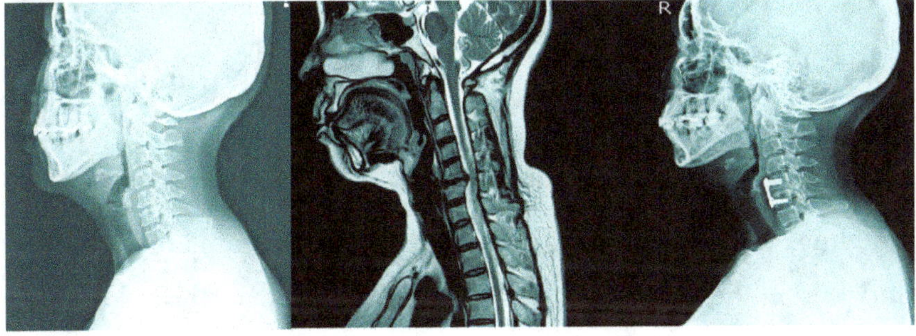

11) At least twenty-one days must elapse before an EMG/NCV is performed. **TRUE**

One of the most common electro diagnostic tests utilized to determine if nerves have been injured is a test called an EMG/NCV. One must wait two to three weeks after a nerve injury to assess the nerve to see if it's been injured. The reason for this is that a process called Wallerian Degeneration must occur first and be complete for a positive test to be present. This process is dependent on how long the nerve axon is. The longer the axon (nerve) is, the longer the process will take. However, the more seriously the nerve is injured, the faster this degeneration and thus the quicker a positive result on an EMG/NCV test will appear.

So if you have people who have suffered trauma with any of the following:

Tingling, numbness, muscle weakness, muscle pain, or cramping and pain in the extremities, an EMG/NCV may be performed after careful clinical examination, to pinpoint the level of nerve pressure and subsequent pathology.

If you have already performed and EMG/NCV test and the results were negative, the test may have been done soon before Wallerian Degeneration was complete. Especially if the patient's symptoms are the same or have gotten worse.

Nerve injury can also cause problems with digestion, urination, respiration and circulation.

Repeat EMG/NCV testing can also be beneficial in determining the amount of neurological recovery after a period of time. Sometimes the nerves recover and sometimes they do not.

(Feinberg J MD, MS: "EMG: Myths and Facts", HSS J 2006 Feb 2(1): 19-21)

12) After a spinal nerve root is compressed by a herniated disc, muscle weakness occurs before numbness develops. FALSE

The anatomy of the spinal nerve root is as follows. If the spinal nerve root is cut in cross section, the fibers in the outside of the nerve root are the sensory nerves. The fibers on the inside of the nerve root are the motor nerves.

Sensory nerves carry information, or nerve impulses from the sensory receptors in our body located in our skin, muscles, joints, etc. up to the brain to let us know what is in our environment. Examples would be cold, heat, pain, and vibration. So the information travels from the outside up to the brain.

Motor nerves carry impulses from our brains to our muscles to make our body move in certain ways. So for example, if we want to flex the biceps, an impulse starts in the brain, travels down the spinal cord and out a spinal nerve root in the cervical spine (neck), down the arm to the biceps muscle to make it contract. This same action occurs for actions such as breathing and digestion (contraction of smooth muscle in surrounding the digestive organs and any muscle containing anatomical structure in the body.)

This continual system of receiving information from the environment and reacting to the environment with motor nerves is how we get by every day with monitoring and adjustments every microsecond.

So if a herniated disc puts pressure on a spinal nerve root after trauma, the first structures of the nerve root that will have pressure is the outer portion of the nerve root which contains the sensory fibers. This will give the person a sensory feeling. It may be pain, numbness, or even feeling heat, cold, or vibration.

The motor nerves which are in the inside of the spinal nerve root are affected much later after time and prolonged pressure on the nerve root causing Wallerian degeneration which I've mentioned in previous articles which is why EMG/NCV testing must be done three to four weeks after trauma.
(Kaiser JT, Lugo-Pico J: National Library of Medicine, Neuroanatomy, Spinal nerves

Feinberg JMD,MS: "EMG: Myths and Facts", HSS J 2006 Feb 2(1): 19-21)

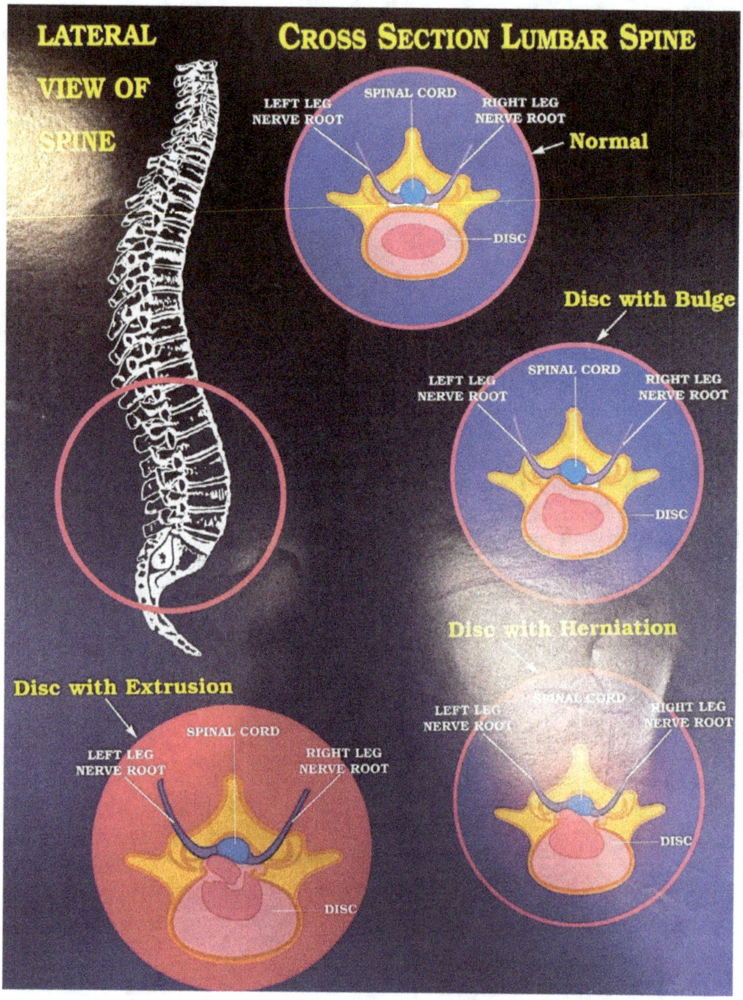

Cross Section of a Spinal Nerve Root

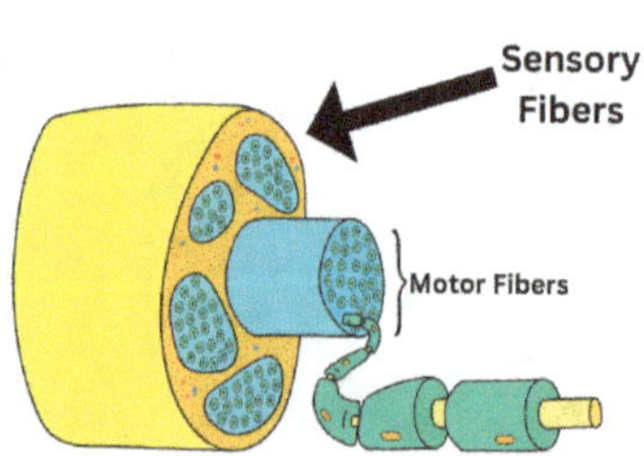

13) A stand-up **MRI** study will always show the same result as a laying down **MRI. FALSE**

The pressure on the lumbar spine is as following:

Laying down on your back: 25 mm mercury pressure

Laying on your stomach: 75 mm mercury pressure

Standing: 100 mm mercury pressure

Standing bent forward: 150 mm mercury pressure

Standing bent more forward: 220 mm mercury pressure

Sitting: 140 mm mercury pressure

Sitting slouched forward: 185 mm mercury pressure

Sitting slouched more forward: 275 mm mercury pressure

So as can be seen above, the position the patient is directly related to the amount of pressure that is exerted on the lumbar discs. This is the reason that most people with disc herniations have most of their pain while seated, less pain when they get up and walk around and the least amount of pain while lying down.

So it is important to realize that an **MRI** study result lying down may yield a disc herniation result which is less severe than the same study performed while seated. This is very important to keep in mind. A person may also have a normal **MRI** while laying down, with just tears in the disc fibers (annulus) but when they go to standing or sitting the disc can be seen to herniate out of position and thus cause spinal nerve root pressure.

This is the reason why **MRIs** are now being done in flexion and extension so we can also see the effects of this changing posture on the disc herniation.

After all, our injured patients are constantly moving all day, and these discs are continuously moving in and out of place or getting bigger and smaller.

(Ergonomic Trends: Back and Disc Pressure in different positions chart Body positions affecting the spine and discs, everything you need to know, Nabil Ebraheim, MD

The effects of standing & different positions on lumbar lordosis: Radiographic studies of 30 healthy volunteers: 11 Youp Cho, Si Young Park, Jong Hoon Park, Tae Kwan Kim, Tae Wan Jung, Hyun Min Lee, Asian Spine- 2015 Oct 9(5)762-769)

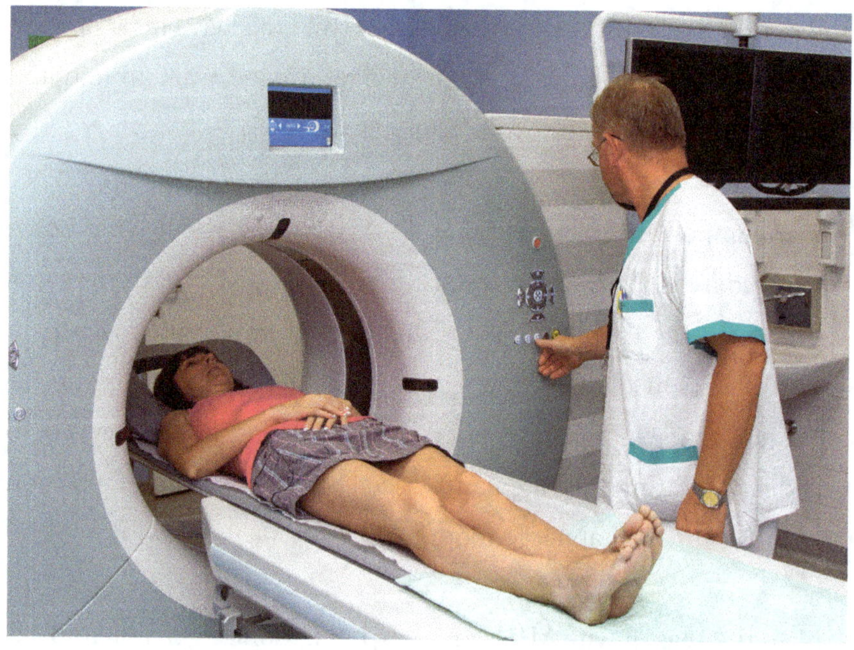

14) You must wait at least thirty days before an MRI is performed after a motor vehicle accident. FALSE

This is a myth that has been around for a long time. After a trauma, if a disc or soft tissue around the disc is injured, the damage such as a tear or a disc herniation is immediate. This would be the same thing as saying that if a patient fractures a bone we must wait thirty days before we do an x ray.

In order for a health care provider to make an accurate diagnosis and render the best treatment possible to a patient, he/she must have the information that is needed to make an accurate diagnosis and when treating the patient but always, "First do no harm."

If a patient after an accident has a clinical exam which indicates that there's a good chance that his/her patient may have a fracture, an x ray must be ordered to determine if the bone is indeed fractured, after which the appropriate treatment is rendered. Would a doctor begin physical therapy on a patient with a fracture, or make sure that a fracture is not present before beginning? Likewise, if after a clinical exam, it is indicated that the patient may have disc pathology and/or ligamentous injury, an MRI must be ordered to determine if the patient has pathology. In my opinion, if treatment is begun without having this information, the patient is at risk for treatment that may be contraindicated or dangerous. Remember, "First do no Harm."

Yogesh Kumar and Daichi Hayashi stated, "Ideally MRI should be performed within seventy-two hours of injury as the T2 hyperintensity produced by edema improves the conspicuity of the ligaments which are seen as low signal intensity in normal state [9]. Later on, resolution of the edema and hemorrhage reduces sensitivity of MRI to detect ligamentous injuries. So actually waiting decreases the sensitivity of the MRI study. You may not even see the ligament injury because you waited too long after the trauma to do an MRI. Now you have a normal MRI and you begin treatment without knowing that there are damaged ligaments in the area that you are working on."

As a doctor of chiropractic, I want to make sure that I have the best diagnostic information possible, before I put my hands on my patient's spine or other body parts and begin to render treatment. Other health care professionals should also require this information. To me, anything less may be considered malpractice.

(Yogesh Kumar, Daichi Hayashi: BMC Musculoskeletal Disorders 2016; 17:310)

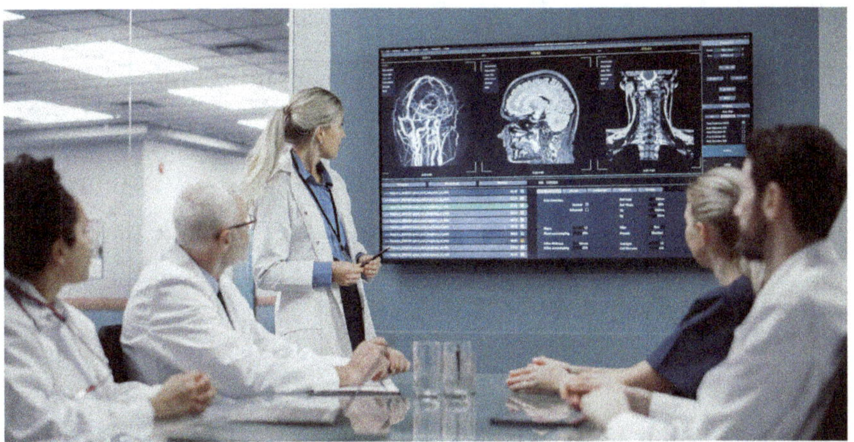

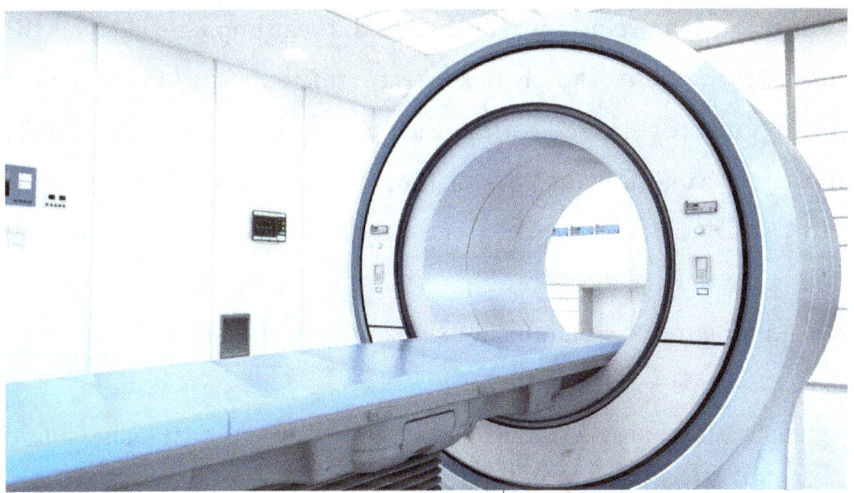

15) An infant seated in an infant car seat facing backwards has a low chance of developing a neck injury in a rear end collision. FALSE

Although the American Academy of Pediatrics has recommended since 2011 that children under two years of age sit in the rear seat of the car in a car seat facing backwards, there are twelve states that recommend that children sit rear facing until the age of one.

When an infant is sitting backward in the rear seat of a motor vehicle, and the vehicle is rear ended, the rear impact will cause the infant's neck to first rapidly flex forward (the opposite of a passenger facing forward) and then when the vehicle comes to a stop rapidly move back smashing the back of the infant seat. Car seats sold in the USA must meet crashworthiness requirements only for frontal collisions. The National Highway Traffic Safety Administration is considering new regulations for side and rear impacts.

When crash dummy tests have been performed with rear facing infant seats, it has been noted that sometimes after rear impact, the car seat can actually rotate forward, causing the infant's head to smash against the rear seat, and then rebound back into its normal position. When the first responders arrive they usually find an infant with a car seat in its normal position accompanied by a screaming infant.

A study published in the October Journal of Traffic Injury Prevention, found that an infant-sized crash-test dummy registered serious head injuries when its rear-facing car seat pitched forward toward the back of the vehicle-in rear end crash tests. Test videos show the top of the car seat and the dummy's exposed head being thrown into the back of the vehicle seat in which the car seat was attached. The estimated head injuries were more severe, the study found, when the car seat was attached via the vehicle seat's lower "LATCH" anchors compared with seat belts.

"It's basic physics" in a rear-end collision, said Jamie Williams, one of the study's authors and a biomedical engineer for Robson Forensic, a Lancaster, Pennsylvania, firm that provides expert witness testimony in lawsuits, including car crashes. "It shouldn't be a surprise to anyone. The only surprise was the magnitude of the head strikes. We didn't think it would be that bad."

A baby's neck muscles are fairly weak when they're born. If you pull them up gently by their hands into a sitting position their head will flop back because their neck muscles can't support it. For the first few months, they'll rely on you using your hands to support their head and neck when you hold them.

Children are, in fact, more susceptible to whiplash because their heads are often not proportionate to their body because their body is still growing. The weight of their head can continue moving forward after the rear end collision, and then when the vehicle stops, it will smash backward against the seat or car seat.

Research shows that even infants are affected by and can remember events that threaten their sense of safety. A response such as PTSD following a traumatic event is not about the event itself, it is a result of the perception of powerlessness.

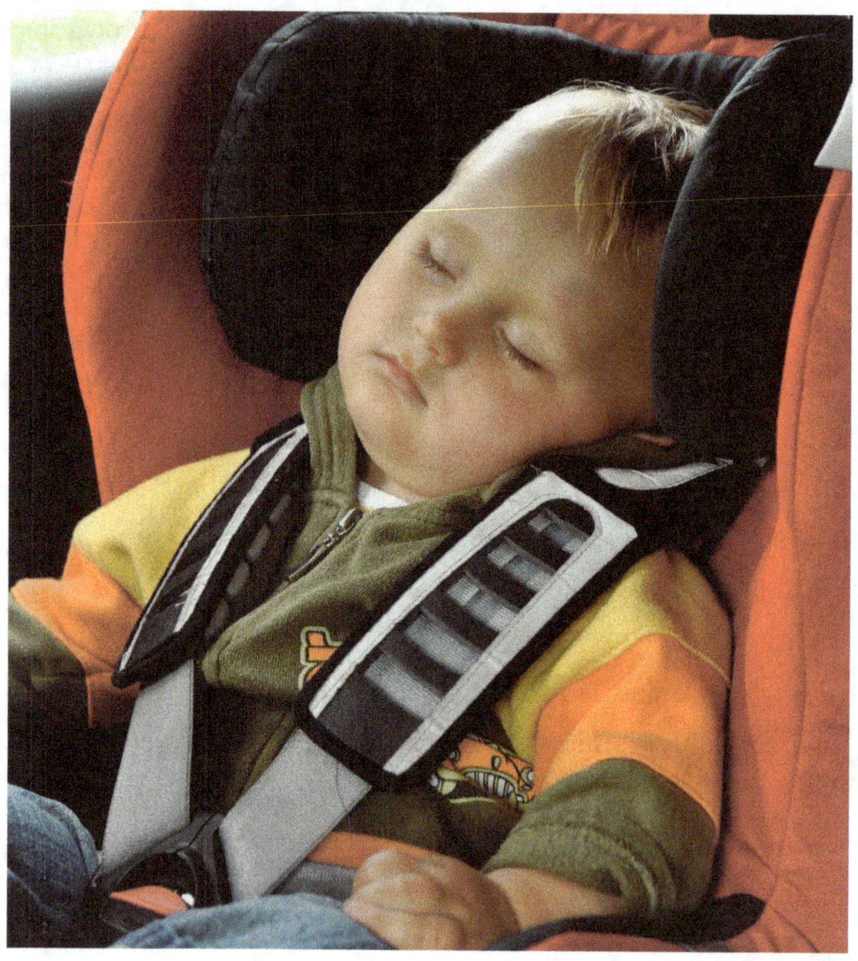

Because infants and young toddlers can't speak, they can't tell doctors that their head hurts or they feel nauseated: symptoms of a potentially serious concussion. She said studies show that early childhood head injuries often don't become apparent until a child starts school. By then, she said parents, doctors and teachers might not link cognitive problems to a traffic crash several years earlier.

It is still highly recommended that infants remain in the back seat facing backward because Trowbridge said regulations focus on front end collisions because they account for about forty-three percent of injuries to children in car seats. Side impact crashes account for about thirty-three percent and rear end crashes nine percent.

I wonder if these numbers are incorrect because the damage to infants in rear end collisions may be overlooked and symptoms may not develop for years.

In any case, always have your infant examined by a qualified health care professional after a motor vehicle accident, even if they are in an infant car seat.

(Williams, Journal of traffic injury prevention, October 2015, Rear facing car seats.

Katherine Shaver, Washington Post, Nov 2015, Study of rear end crashes finds head injuries from rear facing seats.

New York Times, Nov 18, 2015, Keep that child seat facing to the rear.)

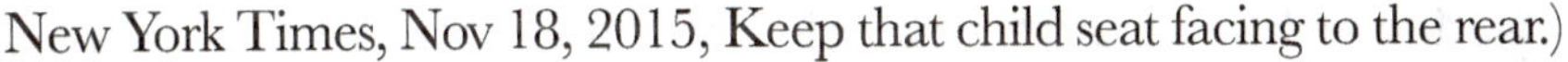

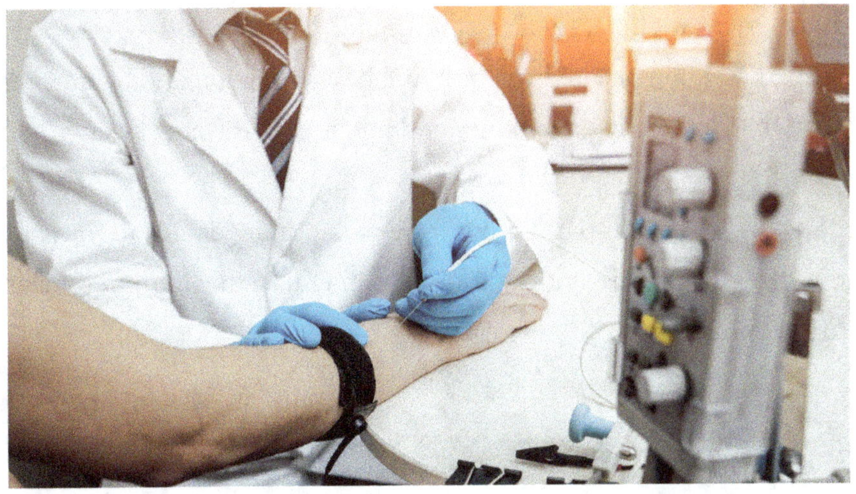

16) If an occupant sees the rear end collision about to happen in his/her rear-view mirror, the best thing to do is to lean forward away from the seatback and reach across to hold his/her child against the seat back of the child's seat. **FALSE**

The worst thing a driver or occupant can do, if they know they're about to be rear ended, is to lean forward away from the back rest. The closer your body is to the back rest and headrest, the less backward occupant movement after rear end collision. If the driver is away from the seat, after rear impact they will rapidly accelerate backward toward the seat and suffer a tremendous whiplash injury and other injuries as well. So if you see a rear end collision about to happen to your vehicle, press your back and head against the seat back and headrest. (Remember the headrest should be placed slightly above the head for maximal protection and not directly behind the head because of ramping)

As far as reaching for a child to help them, if you see a rear end collision about to happen, this will do nothing but cause further cause injury to your shoulder, arm, and hand. If your child's car seat is properly set up, the child will have the best protection and by moving your child, you may move your child into a less protected position.

PS) This is why it is paramount for an examining doctor to find out these details to fully understand what may have been injured prior to examination.

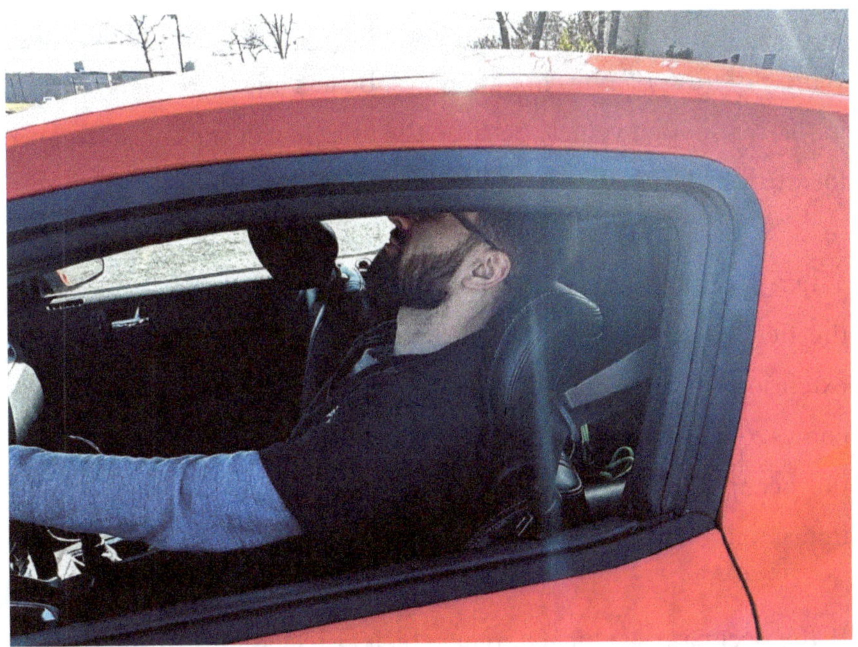

(Nygren A: Injuries to car occupants-some aspects of interior safety of cars. Acta-oto- laryngologica (suppl. #394), 1984

Severy DM, Mathewson JH, Bechtol CP: Controlled automobile rewr-end collisions, an investigation of related engineering & mechanical phenomenon. Can Services Med J 11: 727, 1955

Mertz HJ. Jr., Patrick LM. Investigation of the kinematics & kinetics of whiplash. IN: Proceedings, 111th Stapp Car Crash Conference, SAE 70919

https://dmv-practice-test.com/question/if-you-are-about-to-be-hit-from-the-rear-you-should-not-bnjnnso)

17) If, after a rear end collision, the vehicle being struck hits another vehicle in front of him/her, there will be less injury to the occupants in the rear ended vehicle because the vehicle will travel less distance forward. **FALSE**

When a vehicle is rear ended, the occupant slides up the seat and the head is rapidly extended backward over the headrest (hyper-extension) and then as the vehicle moves forward and eventually comes to a stop, the slower this forward deceleration, the less rapidly the occupant's head moves forward, and the less forward flexion injury to the neck.

If the occupant's vehicle (target vehicle) accelerates forward rapidly and then comes to a stop rapidly, the occupant's head moves forward very rapidly and flies forward into hyper flexion. This causes a serious whiplash (acceleration/deceleration) injury.

In other types of collisions, say a T-bone collision (side-impact collision), if the driver's side is hit, the driver's head will laterally flex to the left toward the driver's side window and strike it. If the vehicle continues to move sideways after impact (let's say it's an icy road) the head will not bounce off the window rapidly into right lateral flexion. If the road is dry, or the vehicle which is T-boned strikes another vehicle on the passenger's side, the vehicle will slide to the right and stop even faster potentially causing more acceleration of the driver's head to the right and even more neck damage.

It is extremely important for both the health care practitioners and the attorneys to understand these types of crash dynamics to truly understand how the injuries to the occupants of vehicles occur.

(Severy DM, Mathewson JH, Bechol CP: Controlled Automobile rear-end collsions-an investigation of related engineering and medical phenomenon. In: Medical Aspects of Traffic Accidents Proceedings of the Montreal Conference, 1955, pp 152-184

Mertz HJ Jr., Patrick LM: Investigation of the kinematics of whiplash. IN: Proceedings, 11th Stapp Car Crash Conference, SAE 670919. Detroit, MI Society of Automotive Engineers, 1967

Foreman SH, Croft AC: Whiplash Injuries: The Cervical Acceleration/Deceleration Syndrome. Baltimore, Williams & Wilkins, 1988, p 66)

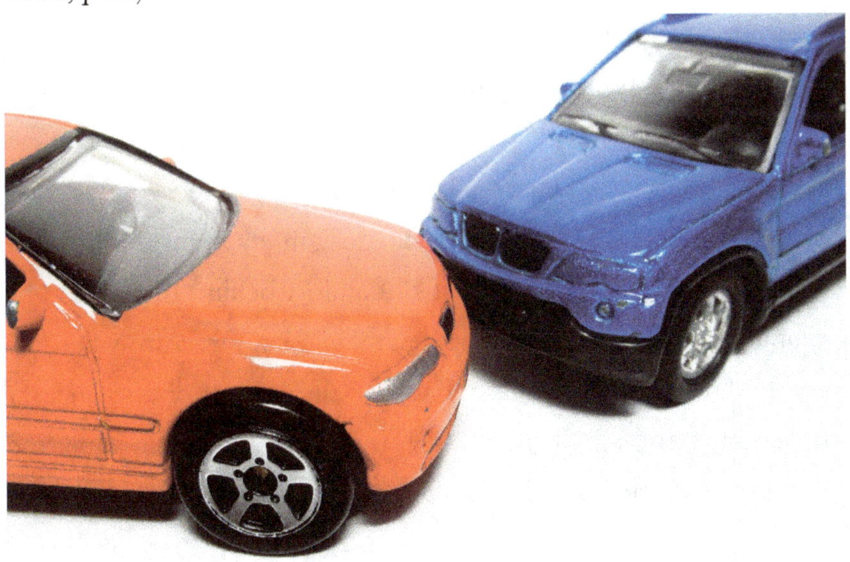

18) Seatbelts prevent all injuries in a rear end collision.　FALSE

Statistics show that seatbelts prevent the person from being thrown through the windshield and in to the steering wheel. It also has been shown that those that wear seatbelts are less likely to die. According to the NHTSA, seat belts reduce the risk of death by 45% and cut the risk of serious injury by 50%. But seat belts also can cause injury. Also, according to the National Highway Traffic Safety Administration NHTSA, thousands of people suffer severe injuries or lose their lives every year due to a defective or malfunctioning seatbelt. Statistics and facts show that approximately three million people are injured annually because of a seat belt failure.

Other types of injuries are created by seatbelts. A very common injury is injuries to the knees. In a rear end collision, after the occupant is thrown back and then forward it is quite common for the occupant's knees to hit the dashboard. The seatbelt holds the abdomen, but the lower part of the body and pelvis can slide forward under the lap part of the belt allowing the knee or knees to strike the dashboard. Once the knees strike the dashboard, this compression can cause posterior cruciate ligament injury which the occupant usually feels as pain or discomfort behind the knee. The occupant can also experience patella (knee cap) fracture when the knee or knees strike the dashboard. If the impact of the knee or knees is hard enough, it can cause compression of the hip joints and hip joint injury such as labral tears and other hip soft tissue injuries.

As mentioned in previous articles, shoulder injuries can also occur as well as vertebral fractures.

Rutledge R, Thomason M, Oller D, Meredith W, Moylan J, Clancy T, Cunningham P, Baker C: The spectrum of abdominal injuries associated with the use of seat belts. J Trauma 31(6): 820-826, 1991.

Asbun HJ, Irani H, Roe EJ, Bloch JH: Intra-abdominal seat belt injury. J Trauma 30(2): 189-193, 1990

Patel, MS, Quereshi AA, Green TP, Dashboard Knee, Surg Engl, 2015 March ;97(2)

Alaia MJ, Posterior Cruciate Ligament (PCL) Injuries, Oct 2021, Ortho Info-Diseases & Conditions

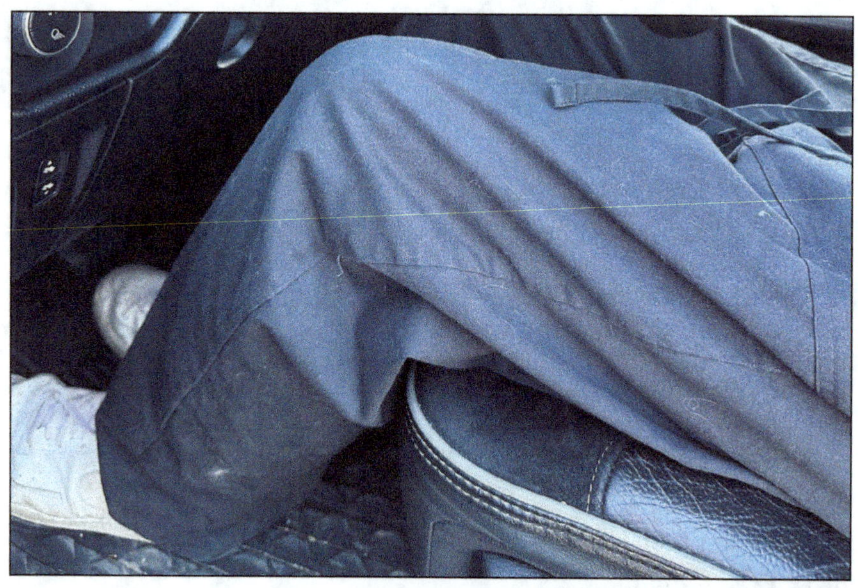

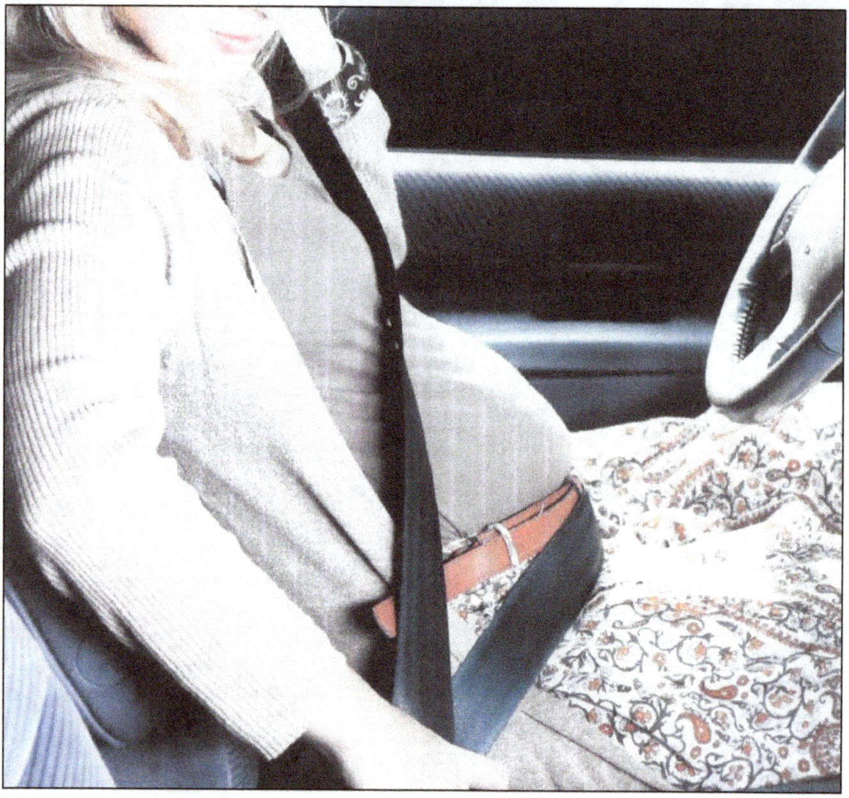

19) A rear seat lap belt harness can cause lumbar spine fractures. **TRUE**

If the rear seat passenger has only a lap belt (two-point restraint system), the risk of lumbar spine fracture is greater than if the rear seat passenger has a three-point restraint system. The reason for this is that in a rear end collision after the occupant moves backward and moves up the seat back, when the vehicle comes to a stop, the occupant is thrown forward and the lap belt stops the occupant from moving forward by squeezing the abdomen and thus pushing back against the front of the lumbar spine, causing the lumbar spine to be bent at an acute angle forward. This acute angle can fracture the vertebrae behind the seat belt and rupture discs or ligaments that hold these vertebrae in place. With higher speed collisions, fractures and then dislocations can occur.

If a rear seated occupant is wearing a three-restraint seat belt, their forward motion will not be as far, but because only 1 shoulder is restrained, as they move forward twisting and torquing of the lumbar spine will occur. This motion can easily cause disc and other lumbar soft tissue injury as well as abdominal injury.

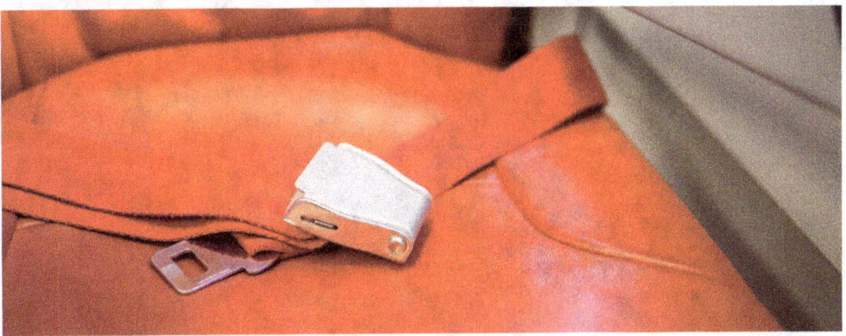

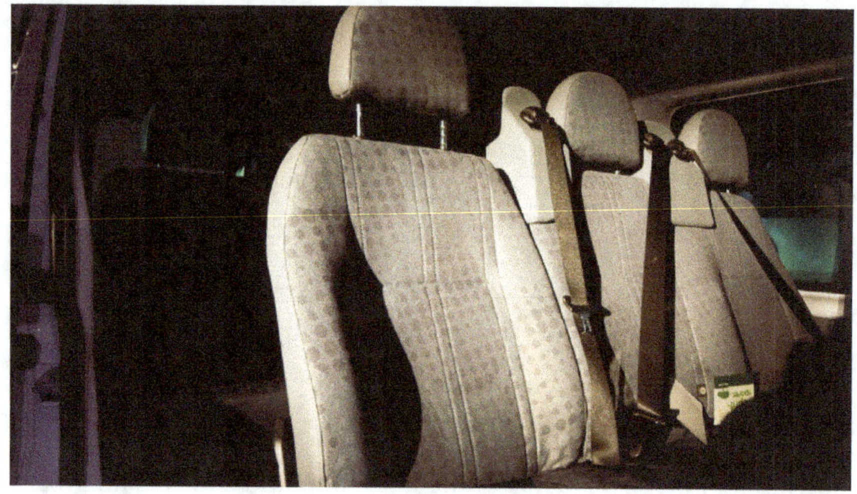

(Holt BW: Spines and Seat belts: mechanisms of spinal injury in motor vehicle crashes. Med J Austral 2:411-413, 1976

Johnson DL, Falci S: The diagnosis and treatment of pediatric lumbar spine injuries caused by rear seat lap belts. Neurosurg 26(3)434-440,1990.

Huelke D, Kaufer H: Vertebral column injuries and seat belts. J Trauma 15:304-318, 1975)

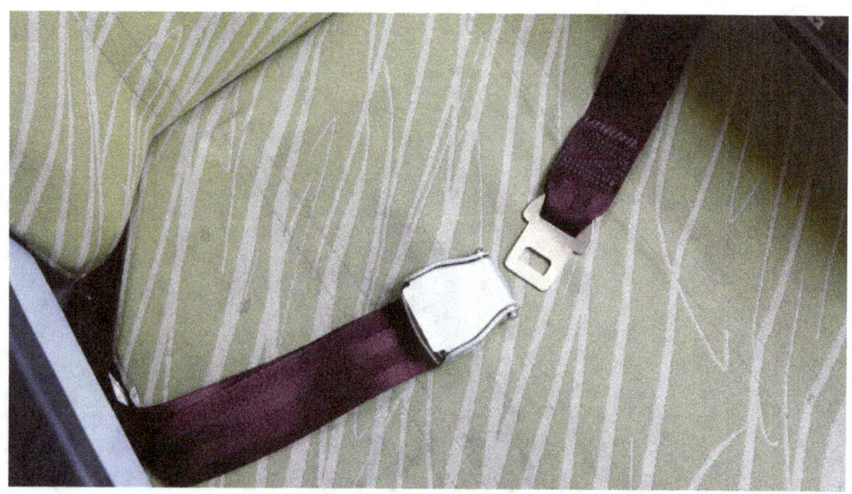

20) Some occupants have suffered from carotid artery dissections and strokes after being rear ended. **TRUE**

The arteries of the neck that carry blood to the brain are the carotid arteries and the vertebral arteries. There is one carotid artery on each side of the neck. After a rear end collision, the occupant's body slides up the seat back (ramping) and then the occupant's head hyper extends backward. When the vehicle comes to a stop or decelerates, the occupant's body slides down the seat and their heads flexes forward rapidly. The three-point seat belt stops the occupant from moving forward in to the steering wheel and windshield. Unfortunately, because only one shoulder is restrained (in the case of the driver the left shoulder and in the case of the front seat passenger the right shoulder) the seat belt can press into the left side of the neck muscles and in some instances to carotid artery on the left and the carotid sinus. The carotid sinus, also known as the carotid bulb, is a neurovascular structure that appears as dilation at the bifurcation of the common carotid artery, and the beginning of the internal carotid artery. If you press on the carotid sinus, you can get bradycardia (slow heart rate), vasodilatation (opening up of blood vessels), and hypotension (low blood pressure). The response is manifested clinically as syncope (fainting or passing out) and has caused fatal results. The same mechanism occurs when a martial artist uses a "sleeper hold" on a person by squeezing their neck with a hold until they pass out. In an article published by Fares Najari and Ali Mohammed Alimomohammadi, "An Immediate Death by seat belt compression; a forensic report," it was found that a forty-nine year old man without any co morbidities dies from compression of the carotid sinus by a seatbelt in a rear end collision. In this same article, the authors noted that with femoral belts in rear seats of cars (two-point system /lap belt only) improper use of this belt could also lead to soft tissue injuries and even small bowel perforation and rupture of solid organs. With damage to the small intestine and colon and lumbar spine. The authors called this "safety belt syndrome."

Three-point restraint systems have also lead to fractures of the ribs, sternum, clavicle, and neck vertebrae. With severe accidents, rupture of the aorta and ventricle of the heart have also occurred.

(Hart RG, Easton JD: Dissections of cervical and cerebral arteries. Neurol Clin 155-182. 1983

Najari F, Mohammed Alimohammadi A: An Immediate Death by Seat Belt Compression; a Forensic Medicine Report: Emerg (Tehran) v.3(4), Autumn 2015)

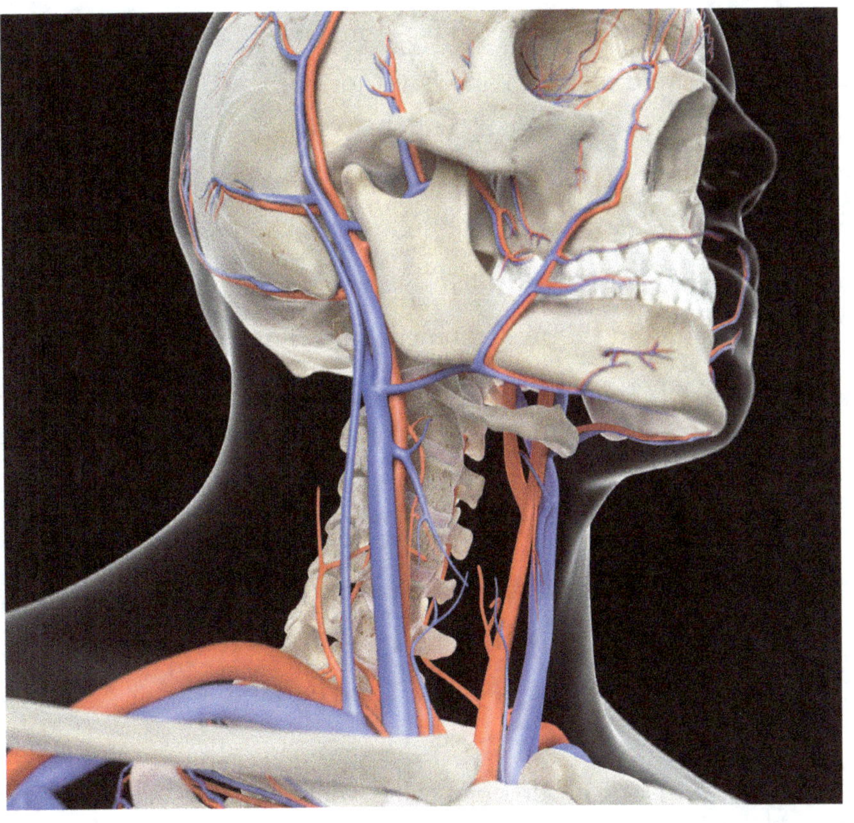

21) A whiplash victim can suffer from neck pain which radiates down the arm to the hand and have normal x ray findings, normal MRI findings and a positive EMG/NCV exam showing a radiculopathy. TRUE

If a person has a vertebra which has been traumatically knocked out of alignment, and this misalignment causes pressure on one of the exiting spinal nerve roots the following can occur. Chemical changes start to occur around the soft tissues of the nerve root causing inflammation and swelling. The vertebral segment now is stuck in the wrong position and does not move back in to place on its own. As this swelling and inflammation continues to get worse, the exiting nerve root starts to function abnormally in which the patient may feel numbness or tingling in the arm and or hand.

This whole situation described above is what occurs when a "vertebral subluxation" occurs. If an EMG/NCV is performed on this patient it will probably yield a positive result for a radiculopathy.

So traumatic misalignment (subluxation) may by itself cause radiculopathy or nerve damage.

These vertebral subluxations can also exert pressure on parts of the spinal nerve roots that travel to organs in the body. Abnormal nerve flow due to subluxation can cause symptoms such as nausea vomiting, stomach pain, indigestion, difficulty breathing, difficulty with bowel movements and urination, and sexual dysfunction.

(Gayral L, Neuwirth E.: Clinical Manifestations of the Autonomic Nervous System- Sequential to Osteoarthritis of the Cervical Spine. Lancet, pp 197-198, May 1958

Kunert W- Functional Disorders of the Internal Organs due to vertebral lesions.- Ciba Symposiums, 13(3), 1966

Burke GL: The Etiology & Pathogenesis of Pain of Spinal Origin: Applied Therapeutics, pp 863-867

Schafer DC, PhD, RC- Applied Physiotherapy, Chapter 7: Specific Potentialities of the Subluxation complex.)

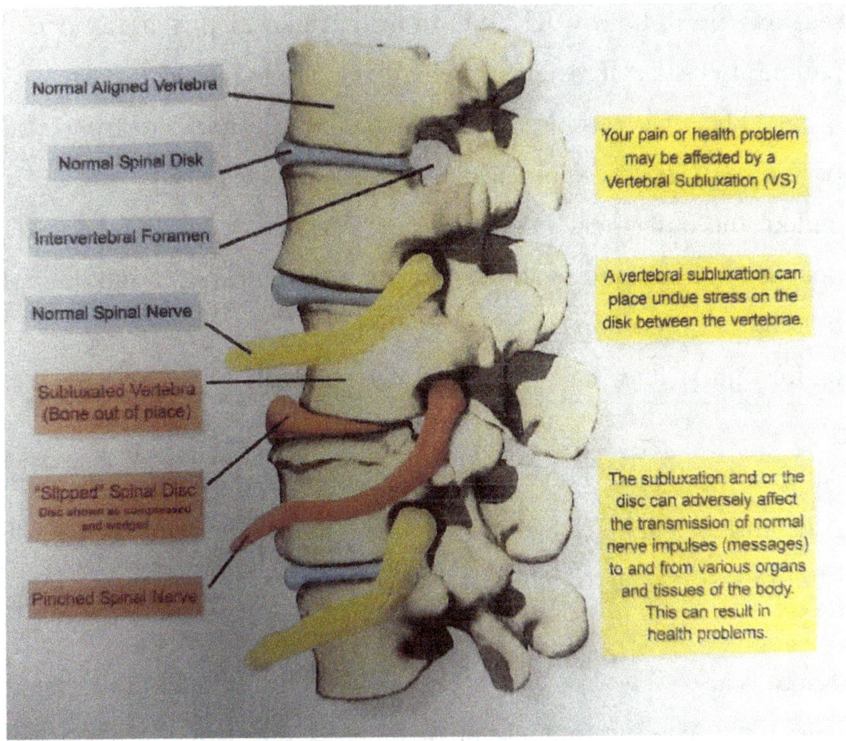

22) A person with a preexisting lumbar disc condition will be injured less than a person without a preexisting lumbar spine condition. FALSE

Most people think that preexisting conditions, such as preexisting herniated discs, lead to less injury after a motor vehicle accident because the discs are already herniated prior to the accident. So how much more new injury could the occupant have?

When I write narrative reports on the injuries of my patients, I refer to preexisting factors as risk factors. Risk factors are physical conditions that exist in the patient prior to the accident that actually set them up to be MORE injured from an accident than a normal patient. Let's take for example two people driving in the front seat of a car. The driver is twenty-five years of age and the front seat passenger is seventy years of age. If this vehicle is stopped and rear ended, the older person will be more seriously injured. The older person's muscles and ligaments are weaker, their discs are more apt to tear, and their bones are not as strong. They have been more set up for injury. They have risk factors.

Attorneys call this "The Eggshell Rule" which states:
A defendant's liability will not be reduced just because the plaintiff is more susceptible to injuries.

There is also "The Eggshell Doctrine" which states that a negligent defendant takes the victim as he or she finds the victim even a victim that is as fragile or delicate as an eggshell.

Another example would be an old osteoporotic woman walking down the street steps in to a hole in the sidewalk, falls, and breaks both legs. This woman had a risk factor called "osteoporosis" (brittle bones) that made her get more injured than a normal person with normal bone density.

Anytime an occupant has arthritis and degeneration in their spines or other joints, these are considered risk factors. These factors will set up this patient for more injury than a person without risk factors.

Anytime an occupant has a previous injury to a joint such as a shoulder, elbow, knee, wrist, hip, ankle, etc., when these joints are subjected to trauma, they will be weaker than normal tissue that had not been injured so there will be more injury after trauma.

(Ehni G: Degenerative motion segment encroachments. In: Cervical Arthrosis: Diseases of the Cervical Motion Segments. Chicago, Year Book, 1984 p 54 en.wikipedia.org/wiki/Eggshell_skull https://en.wikipedia.org/wiki/Eggshell skull)

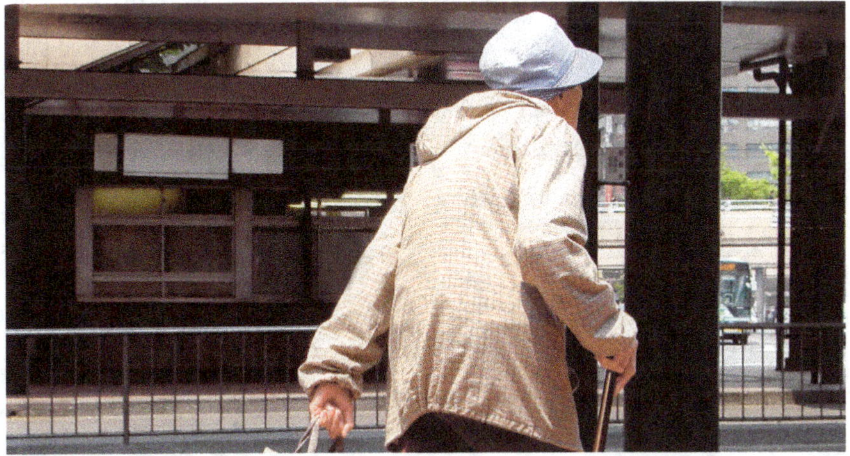

23) In general fractures cause much more long-term effects than sprains. FALSE

When lecturing to doctors and attorneys over many years regarding soft tissue injury, I always ask the audience the following question.

If you've ever broken a bone, please raise your hand. Let's say fifteen hands go up. I then ask this group to please raise your hand again if they still have pain, weakness, or any other kind of symptom as a result of the fracture. Maybe one or two hands are raised if any.

I then ask the audience to please raise your hand if you've ever had a sprain/strain in a part of your body. About thirty hands go up. I then ask the same group to raise their hand again if they still have pain, weakness, or any other kind of symptom in the body part that they sprained or strained. Almost all of the hands are raised back up.

The reason for this is because "fractures usually heal as good as new, and sometimes stronger."
When bones heal, calcium is laid down around the fracture site and usually a callous (ball) of calcium is formed around the fracture site. This usually is so strong after it heals that if in the future another trauma occurs to the same area, a different part of the bone will fracture and not the callous area.

When Tai fighters train, they will take their shin bones and strike trees and or metal poles to create micro fractures in the bone so that calcium and callous formation occurs at the point of impact on their leg. After the shin heals, they will do it again, let it heal, again, let it heal, and again, until eventually they have a big ball of calcium on their shin. Now when they strike an opponent with their shin, it's like getting hit with a sledgehammer.

Soft tissue injuries involve ligaments, tendons, discs, and muscles. Discs, ligaments, and muscles have a very poor blood supply so when they are injured it is very difficult for them to heal and they never return back to normal. Imagine a rubber band that gets stretched out. Some of the rubber fibers must tear for it to get stretched out and it never can return to its normal length again. This loosening of the supporting elements of a joint creates instability or laxity and weakness of the joint which will make it prone to reinjury (risk factor).

So after explaining this, I ask my audience of personal injury attorneys, "Why do you prefer to have injured clients with fractures over those who have soft tissue injuries?"

The answer is that fractures are easy to see, document, and thus prove, where soft tissue injuries traditionally have been difficult to see and document.

With today's technology, it's easier to document and see these soft tissue injuries. With the knowledge that we have about the long-term effects of these injuries that I have presented in my articles it can be clearly seen that soft tissue injuries cause much more serious injuries and much longer effects than fractures most of the time. Of course, there are some fractures that will cause devastating injuries and severe long-term effects or even death, but most of the time this is not the case.

Soft tissue injuries then usually produce much more and longer lasting pain and suffering for the injured person which is often permanent.

According to investigators Dr. Gargan & Bannister report, after ten years, only twelve percent of whiplash victims fully recover. Ian McNab MD reported that of two hundred sixty-six med legal cases of whiplash, forty-five were still symptomatic two years after settlement.

(https://northazrtho.com: Everything you need to know about fractures

McLean A, IN: B.Sc.: 19 Apr 2018-Did You Know

Hammond C, Oct 5, 2018- BBC- Five Myths about Broken Bones)

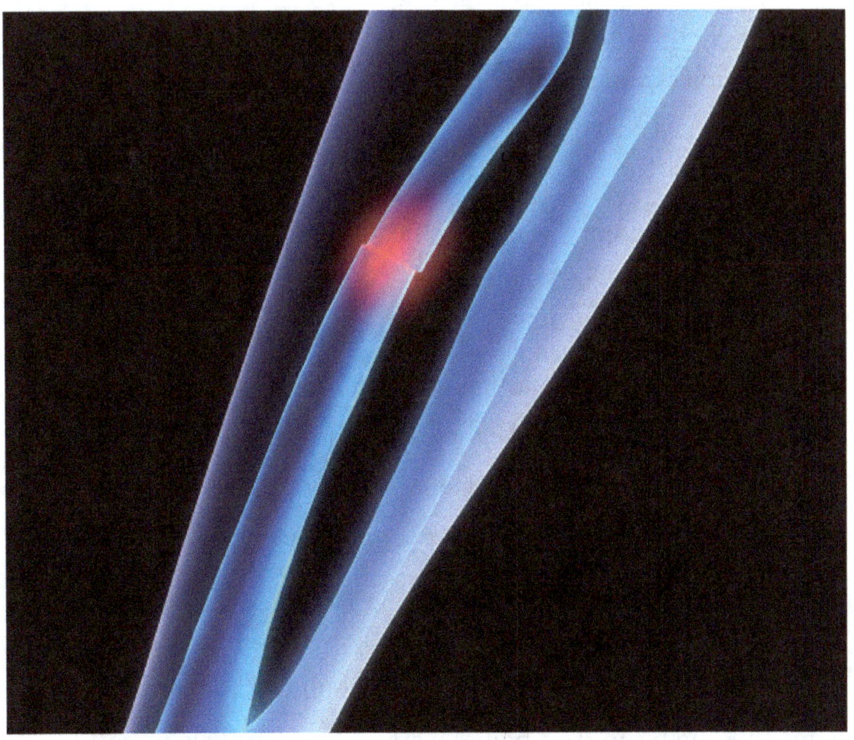

TYPICAL BONE FRACTURES

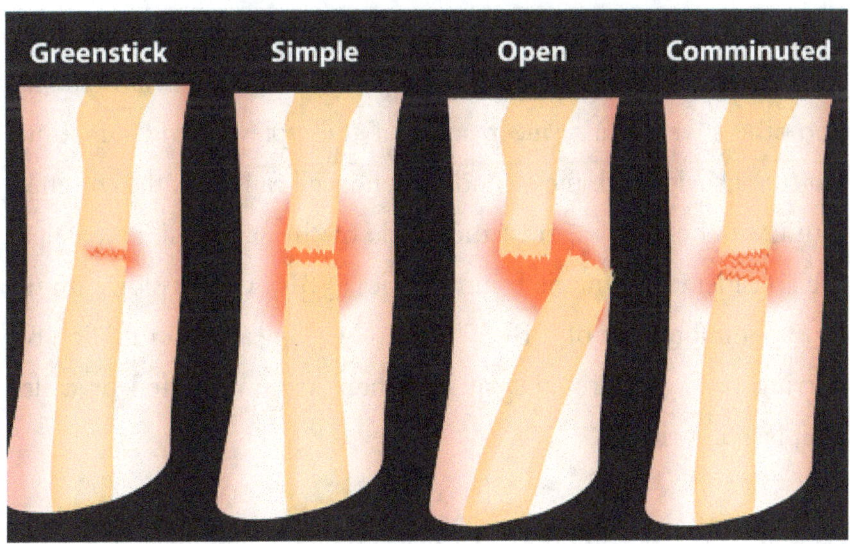

24) You can't get a concussion or traumatic brain injury during an accident unless you strike your head on something inside or outside the vehicle. FALSE

After a whiplash injury, where the head rapidly accelerates backward into hyperextension and then rapidly accelerates forward into flexion serious brain injury and concussion, without any head impact at all can occur. Just imagine putting a water balloon inside of a coconut shell. If we then rapidly shake the coconut, the water balloon will bang around inside the coconut and smash against the inside walls of the coconut and the water balloon may even break inside of the coconut.

In "Shaken Baby Syndrome," the baby is shaken violently and the baby's brain is smashed against the baby's skull on the inside damaging the brain. Football players are constantly getting hit hard and suffering concussions and brain injury. There was a lawsuit made by the NFL players for chronic brain injuries caused by continual concussions which was found to cause a condition called Chronic Traumatic Encephalopathy (CTE). Effects such as dementia and others were the result in some of these players and sometimes violent behavior and suicide and dementia, all caused by the continual hitting of the brain against the inside of the skull. All concussions are considered traumatic brain injuries (TBIs). Concussions are the most common form of TBI. There are up to nearly four million occurring per year. Probably at least half are unreported or called whiplash injuries.

As I have discussed in previous article, even an infant in a car seat can suffer from a concussion without striking the head caused by this rapid movement of the head back and forth. Infant car seats do not prevent this from happening. As a matter of fact, when an infant car seat is faced backward, a rear end collision may cause the seat to rotate forward causing the infant's head to strike the seatback the infant is facing. The seat then rebounds back into its normal position and when the EMTs arrive the baby is crying, unable to say what hurts with the car seat in what appears to be an unmoved position.

With motor vehicle collisions, anything that causes the head of the occupant to move back and forth rapidly could cause the brain to smash on the inside of the skull causing brain injury. This is exactly what happens in a rear end whiplash injury.

Common symptoms of brain trauma or concussion are:

Headache or "pressure" in head, nausea, vomiting, balance problems or dizziness, double or blurry vision, and sensitivity to light and noise.

Authorities say that it takes about ninety to one hundred grams of force to cause a concussion which equates to smashing your skull against the wall at twenty miles per hour. Remember the "2.5-5" rule. The head of the occupant will move backward in a whiplash at two and a half to five times the speed of rear impact. So a five miles per hour rear impact will cause the head to move twelve and a half to twenty-five miles per hour. A ten miles per hour impact will cause the head to move twenty-five to fifty miles per hour. So as you can see, with minor rear end impact, brain injury can occur.

You can also suffer from a post traumatic brain injury without knowing it. Sometimes brain injury symptoms will not happen till weeks later. The occupant may suddenly experience dizziness and headaches and may not remember having the injury. Depression and anxiety may also be caused by TBI (Traumatic Brain Injury).

The long-term effects of whiplash and brain injury can be very serious and can cause tremendous difficulties physically, mentally and in the activities of daily living.

(Hohl M: Soft Tissue injuries of the neck in automobile accident. J Bone Joint Surg 56A(8): 1675-1682, 1974

Brenner C, Friedman A, Merrit HH: Posttraumatic headache. Neurosurgery 1: 370-391, 1944.

Russel WR: Cerebral involvement in head injuries; a study of 200 cases. Brain 55:549, 1932

Denker PG, Perry GF: Postconcussion syndrome in compensation and litigation: analysis of 95 cases with electroencephaagraphic correlations. Neurology 4: 912-918, 1954

Mayo Clinic Family Health Book. Fifth Edition

HTTPS://www.bumc.bu.edu>busm

Handbook of Clinical Neurology, Volume 158, 2018 pp 21-24

Sports Medicine Handbook, 2011-2012 Concussion or mild Traumatic Brain Injury (mTBI) in the Athelete.

Https://www.calendar-canada.ca/faq/how-much-force-does-it-take-to-ger—a-concussion)

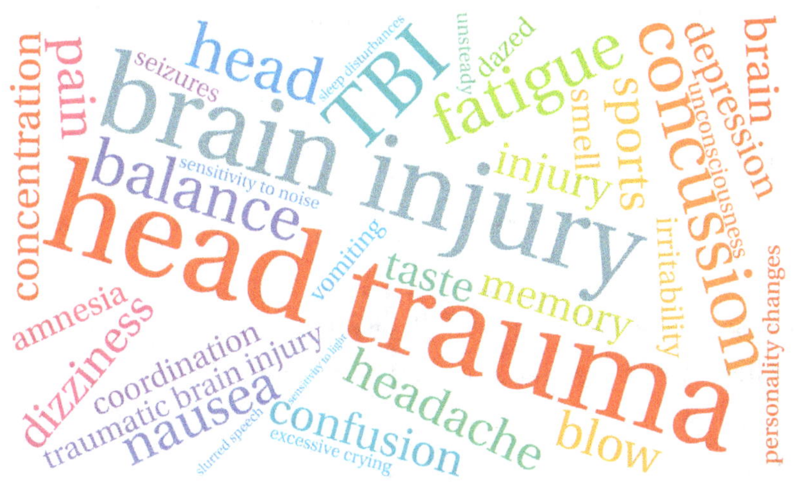

TYPES OF CONCUSSIONS

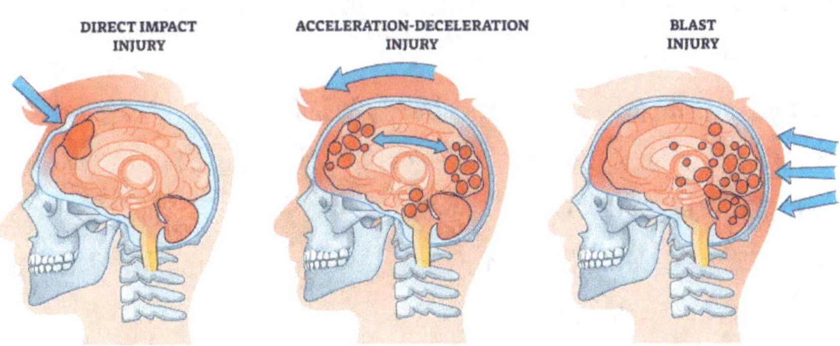

ACCIDENT QUESTIONNAIRE

1. Time and date of the accident:

2. Street and town where accident occurred:

3. Diagram your accident; in the diagram indicate YOUR vehicle as #1 and the other vehicle as #2. Use arrows to indicate direction of each vehicle.

4. Type and weight of your vehicle:

5. Type and weight of other vehicle:

6. Did you have your foot on the brake at the time of impact? Yes No

If Yes, did you take your foot off the brake after impact? Yes No

7. After impact, how far did your vehicle travel?

8. After impact, in what direction did your vehicle travel?

9. Was your seat belt fastened? Yes No

10. Is there a shoulder harness with your seat belt? Yes No

11. Was your head rest position: Circle one

Behind your head , or above your head, below your neck ,
or behind your neck

12. Did your head hit the windshield? Yes No

13. Did your head hit any other window in your car or any other part of the car? Yes No

14. Did your vehicle hit anything else after being hit: another vehicle, structure, or object? Yes No

15. Were there passengers in your vehicle? Yes No

16. What symptoms or complaints did you have immediately after

the accident?

17. What symptoms or complaints do you have now?

18. Were the police notified? Yes No

19. Were you taken to the hospital? Yes No

20. If the answer to #20 was yes, how did you get there, by ambulance or car?

21. Were you employed before the accident? Yes No

22. Since the accident, have you been able to return to work? Yes No

23. Have any doctors examined you since the accident? Yes No If so, please list their names and addresses:

24. Were any pictures taken of your vehicle after the accident? Yes No If so, please send a copy to this office.

25. Did you have any bruises, cuts, or abrasions as a result of this accident? Yes No

26. If the answer to #25 is yes, were pictures taken? Yes No If so, please send copies to this office. If no pictures were taken and it is still possible to see the injuries, please take pictures .